SEEKING THE SUN THROUGH THE

Storm

The Stroke That Saved My Life

By Donnie Edison

Seeking The Sun Through The Storm

The Stroke That Saved My Life

ISBN-13: 978-0-578-82645-5

Dedication

NATALIA EDISON
GARY RUNGO
DENNIS ROGERS
AMIR & FLO (my dad and mom)
THOMAS EDISON (my brother, not the inventor)
Without these amazing souls I don't know where I'd be.

Acknowledgements

I could not be more grateful for my tribe, most of whom do not share my DNA. Florence and Seyed Mahmood Amir, Monica Amir-Blake and Joe Blake, and the rest of their family, Mark and Mercedes Deams who have treated me like family from the moment I met them. My siblings, Tom, Brad, Lisa, and their families. My late parents, Joe and Sharon Edison. Coach Rungo, and all of the players that I coached at Arlington High School, Dennis Rogers who gave me a playbook for baseball and life, my professors and tutors at RCC and Cal-State San Bernardino.

Austin for showing me true courage and Amarleono Burnett. The Tavaglione Family (George, Angie, and Dawn) for their support, and Natalia Edison.

Foreword

It's not what happens to us in this life, it's how we respond. The day I met Donnie Edison, I knew he had a great lens on his eye. He was a classmate of mine during undergrad, and on the first day of my Mindful Meditation course, in walks Donnie with that unique walk of his. It was the type of walk that may have evoked pity from some of the others in the class, but not from me, why? His white tee shirt bore bright red letters in a smooth font that read "Limpin' ain't easy." It made me laugh because I recognized that this man is aware of his situation, but he is not only making the best of it, he's doing it with a great attitude and smile.

I can appreciate the value of a positive attitude, in conjunction with hard work and discipline. As our relationship grew from classmates, to friends, and eventually to family with Donnie, I realized that I had the right attitude; however, what I lacked was the discipline and hard work. The challenges that Donnie Edison has faced and has overcome in his life, from childhood, to where he is today, will astound the majority of those who read about them.

Seeing Donnie accomplish yet another goal constantly reminds me that I need to keep going. He is in that group of friends of mine that reflects where my life will be in the next five, ten, fifteen, and even twenty years. He is a man some may refer to as disabled, but he's also the one who taught me the meaning of "diff-abled," referring to how he can do anything anyone else can do, he just does it differently.

The contents of what you are about to embark on may seem like enough positivity and motivation to make even the most stagnant person you can think of get up and get moving. I believe what you are about to read is only the foundational stages of an incredible life's journey and legacy. A true story of a real underdog, who made difficult decisions in critical times, which ultimately led to some pretty spectacular victories.

In this book you will read about one man's decision to get up and push forward, every time life tried knocking him down. A decision to not wallow in self-pity, but rather to stand up and fight. Donnie has definitely had life throw him some curve balls, but rather than striking out, he's managed to get a good piece of it, and knock it out of the park. It has truly been an honor and pleasure growing from classmates to friends, to eventually family with the author of this book. I was humbled when he asked me to write a foreword for something he's put so much time and effort into. My hope for anyone who reads this is that when you read Donnie's story and how he's done what he's done with the mindset that he's done it with, you will gain a true appreciation for what we as human beings are capable of. Especially when both sides of our brain's work.

Gabriel Robles

Table of Contents

Prologue

Though my lids were barely open, the blinding fluorescent lights engulfed my pupils

Beep, beep

The sound blared into my left ear.

This doesn't look like my room! Where the heck am I?

Beep! Beep!

The sound blared again. I turned left to find out the source of that annoying sound but all I saw was an unfamiliar plain looking wall.

This doesn't feel like home. Where the hell am I?

"Hi Donnie,"

Okay I know that voice.

"Xavier? Where am I? Why are you here?"

"We were asked to visit you to make sure you were okay. You're in ICU at Kaiser.

"What? Why the heck --? Can you please ask the nurse to turn that beep off of level 20? It's so damn loud!"

"Amir is out in the hall talking with the doctor, I'll let them – explain."

I closed my eyes again and was awakened by a knock at the door sometime later.

"Donnie Boy your eyes are open! How are you feeling?"

My eyes focused on my dad.

"Amir? I'm fine but why am I here?"

Doc walked in, "Glad to see your eyes open Donnie. Who is the President?"

"President Barack Obama, of course."

"Great, what's your birthday?"

"June 14, 1973, I'm not drunk. What the heck is wrong doc?"

"It's a long story, and an ambulance will be transferring you to Ballard. It's a physical rehab hospital in San Bernardino. I don't want you to panic when you get up and try to walk and can't. That's all I'll say right now. I don't want to say anymore right now."

"I can't walk?"

The doctor took a breath.

"You may never walk again Mr. Edison."

How was I supposed to respond to that? Up until this moment, my life felt like a fairytale!

The beeping finally stopped, and my eyes began to adjust to those blue fluorescent lights. I looked around the room finally focusing on some familiar faces. I first saw Xavier who was my friend since kindergarten and my fellow alternative rock music lover.

"Xavier! Is that Julie and Jessica behind you?

He nodded but had an extremely worried look on his face.

"Hey ladies I haven't seen you two in years."

We had both known Julie and Jessica since middle school. It was good to see them but strange at the same time.

"Natalia called me and told me they gave you a five percent chance of living. That's why we are all here."

CHAPTER 1

The Tingle

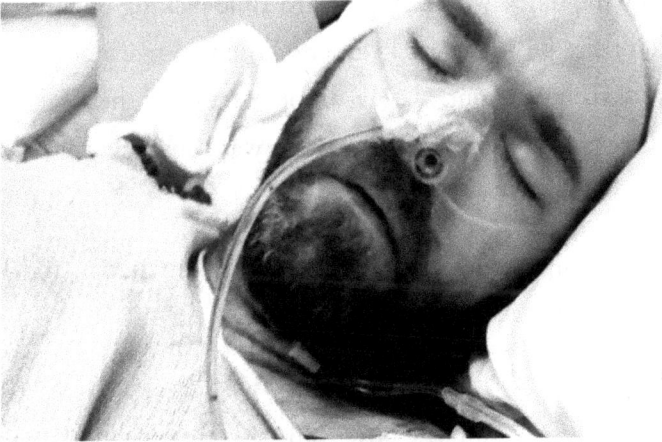

My new wife Natalia and I had been in our new home together for just a few weeks when I started to feel a tingle in my left shoulder while I was at work. I just shrugged it off. It was probably a pinched nerve from tossing my two-year-old niece Callie in the air after a family dinner a few nights before.

But when the numbness had not subsided the next day, I started to really wonder what might be going on. Halfway through tending bar at the restaurant I worked at, I found myself suddenly unable to carry a drink from the beer tap to the bar top. It was almost as if my left hand was completely numb.

"Maybe you're having a stroke,"

Joe was a regular patron and a big talker.

"I'm only 36."

Before that day I only thought elderly people had strokes. *I was too young. Joe must not know what he was talking about.*

But the next day my left arm hit every doorway I walked through, because by that point it seemed like I had no control of it.

What the hell is going on?

The following day, I was having a hard time picking up cinder blocks to build a fire pit in our backyard. So, I figured maybe I really should get my arm checked out. Natalia dropped me off at the local urgent care on her way to pick up Callie who she was babysitting again.

"Donnie Edison!"

After a forty-minute wait, they finally called my name, and I walked into the examination room.

"Hi Doc. I cannot use this left arm much at all."

"Hello Mr. Edison, I am the physician assistant on call."

He asked me a few questions and I told him how I'd tossed my niece in the air and probably pinched a nerve. He asked me to squeeze his hand to test my strength. It was clear that I literally had no strength in my left hand.

He gave me a diagnosis of Brachial Neuritis and sent me to get an x-ray. This rare condition affects the nerves going to the chest, shoulder, arm, and hand. It also causes pain or loss of function in the nerves that carry signals to and from the brain and spinal cord, according to The World Health Organization (WHO).

While I was paying at the window, I found myself laughing uncontrollably when I couldn't seem to get my debit card out of my money clip because of the numbness in my left hand.

When I saw the actual doctor, he verified the Brachial Neuritis diagnosis, but my main concern was why I couldn't use my left hand, and if I ever would be able to again.

"Could this be a stroke?"

The PA shooed me out shaking his head.

"No, No. Claiming, "You're too young."

So I met up with my wife Natalia and niece Callie in the lobby and we were off.

The next morning, on the way to the kitchen to make breakfast, I fell on my face instead. I pushed myself up, but I fell three more times.

"What are you doing?", Natalia asked with a strange look on her face.

"I have no idea."

She immediately looked concerned and walked over to me.

"Try to smile Donnie."

I gave her what I thought was a big grin and she immediately started crying.

I hated to see her so scared.

"It's going to be okay Natalia. Just go get the rolling chair from the office and wheel me to the car."

Natalia zipped me to the ER, and upon arrival, I was immediately given a CT brain scan. Because I was in a semi-conscious state, my family was put in an extremely tough situation, having to make life or death decisions on my behalf. Because my brain was swelling, they had to decide whether or not to let the doctors remove my scalp. This was due to the fact that my brain was pushing up against it with great force.

I was told later that my father-in-law Amir, who is a pretty smart dude, started asking lots of questions. He wanted to know the pros and cons of opening up my scalp, so he would be better able to weigh out the consequences. In the end, he decided that it would not be worth it to remove it. Fortunately, the medication I was given to slow down the swelling, began doing its job.

I vaguely remember going in and out of consciousness and catching glances of my old friends, and Natalia, but not much else. I was aware enough to realize that something serious was going on, but had no idea why I was half-naked and shirtless. At one point, I lifted my hospital gown as if attempting a strip tease.

"You've been waiting years to see this."

I joked with my old high school friend Julie, but she didn't laugh back. Neither did anyone else. There I was trying to lighten the mood just like I'm sure my late Dad would have, but no one was going for it. My nervous and beautiful mother-in-law, Flo Mamma, was right at my side holding my hand with great concern, but at this point I still didn't understand the fuss. Thanks to the meds, I didn't feel any pain and still didn't know what exactly had happened. I just knew I was hungry, but they wouldn't let me eat anything but ice chips.

This was because the function I had lost was still to be determined, and they were not sure how well I was able to swallow. They did have a feeding tube lodged in my nose, but I was more concerned about tasting food than the nutrients. They did their job by being cautious, but I was still very upset that I couldn't eat real food.

I really just wanted to know what the doctors had figured out, and how long it was going to be until I would get to go home and finish building the fire pit. All I could think about was going home with my beautiful wife so we could barbeque outside and enjoy our new life together.

Those thoughts, and a lot more were going through my head after Natalia walked in the room and touched my left hand.

"What happened to me? Why am I here?"

Body language says a lot and her eyes slowly veered away from mine as I waited for her response. She sighed long and heavy.

"It's a long story and I will tell you in a bit, once I get more info from your last brain scan."

Brain scan?

She left, and I drifted off soon after. A while later, she gently woke me up. I didn't like the look on her face because I couldn't tell if I had good or bad news coming my way.

"So how does it look Natalia, do I get to go home soon?"

"Not so fast, Mister,"

The doctor entered with his clipboard.

"The last scan shows that you are missing about 95% of the right side of your brain, so right now you probably can't move your left arm or leg." *This was all caused by a stroke that I had been told I was too young to have!*

"The large blood clot was impeding blood and oxygen from getting to that part of your brain. Without blood, which carries oxygen to the brain, the cells begin to die. When this happens, a person loses whatever function those cells were responsible for. As we all probably know, the brain controls everything we as human beings do:from breathing, to talking, to walking, and everything in between. The exact functions that you lost are still to be determined."

Soon after the brain scan, I was moved into intensive care. That's when Natalia started making phone calls because she was told I had a 5% chance of making it through this alive. I clearly had no idea of the severity of the situation because I was still hardly conscious. The funny thing is if I would have known, I probably would have used that information as motivation. I would have been determined to show those doctors that I was not the typical stroke victim.

I was not a victim at all!

"This can't be true! I'm only thirty-six!" What am I gonna do?"

"I don't know, but we're just going to have to figure it out."

"Am I going to be okay?"

"You will, but your life will definitely be more difficult."

"Are you saying I definitely won't walk again?"

"Well, no, I can't say that, but with all the damage you have to that side of the brain, I will just say. "probably not."

I'm sure you can't possibly imagine what a life altering moment this was for me. No one is immune and unfortunately the way I had lived my life before all this happened, led to this very moment, and I was the only one to blame.

THE TINGLE

When the Doc said that I'd probably never walk again, my initial instinct was to stand up and walk across the room. But when he told me that there was a possibility I would, that's all I needed to hear. I was determined to live out the rest of my days fully, completely, and upright!

I was going to do whatever I had to do, scared as hell or not! I had no idea of the magnitude of what was truly in front of me.

CHAPTER 2

Natalia

As I lay in bed that evening, I began to reflect on the life I had lived. One of the things I was most grateful for was Natalia who just a year prior, had become my wife. We had only just begun building our brand-new life as a married couple in our new home a few weeks ago...

I remembered meeting her on that chilly December night when I had gone to downtown Riverside to get a look at what

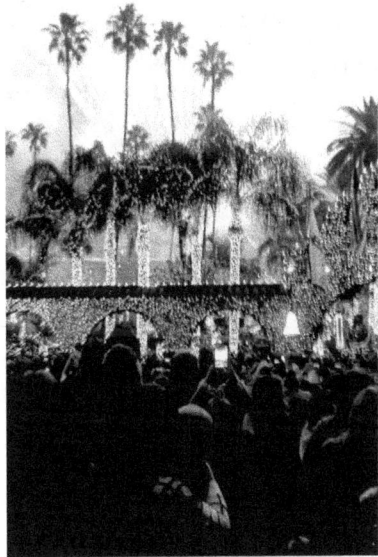

seemed like one million Christmas lights hanging, dangling, and shining brightly on the outside of the well-known historic hotel, The Mission Inn. It was Riverside's version of Rockefeller Center, and it had been a big part of my childhood.

At some point when I had grown tired of feeling like a sardine competing for space on the street with the crowds of other onlookers, I took a detour from the immense display of electrical artwork.

After treating myself to a nice warm dinner at the great local Mexican diner La Cascada, I decided to walk down a few doors to Worthington's. It was the local hole in the wall nicknamed by locals as "The Dub," that mainly Riverside natives knew about. My plan was to warm myself up with a glass of Crown Royal on the rocks, but I got so much more. When I stepped inside, I was immediately captivated by the dark brown eyes of a Hispanic female stranger and my mind started going.

Do I know her? Did I serve her at Friday's?

Stepping out of my comfort zone I eventually made eye contact with her and started coaching myself.

Okay Donnie, don't look over there again until you're ready to go over there.

I kept going back and forth in my mind, and after my last sip of my whiskey, I took a deep breath and approached. I stood in her eye line for just a moment before she noticed me, and I made my move.

"Have I ever served you at the bar at Fridays? You look really familiar."

She responded with a smile that took my breath away.

"I don't think so, what's your name?"

NATALIA

And that was the night I met Natalia. We met at the same place the following week, ordered Newcastles and talked the rest of the night. With her I found an ease I had not felt before with any woman.

She was the manager for her family's popular take-out Mexican restaurant and worked nights. She was very family oriented and when I met her parents it was love at first sight. Amir was a tall Iranian with a heart of gold, and her mother Flo, who I called Flo Mamma, was a beautiful Puerto Rican, who also became an angel to me.

Natalia and I took our time getting to know each other between our schedules and her travels. A year after we met, she took a trip to Europe that she had saved up for. I missed her terribly, and by the time she came back, I knew I no longer wanted to be just her friend.

When she got back in town, I had a surprise lined up for her. I picked her up from the airport wearing a long-sleeved shirt over a short sleeved one. I drove her to her family's restaurant, and we went inside for a bite. Afterwards, I walked her to her car and handed her the sharpie that had been in my outside pocket all along.

"What is this for?"

I unbuttoned my shirt to reveal the t-shirt I was wearing underneath. In silkscreen print it read, "Natalia will you be my girlfriend?" There was a yes and no box for her to check. I looked away, and held my breath, afraid of what her answer would be.

"Donnie, you can look now."

To my great relief, I saw that she had checked the yes box, and I never stopped smiling, even when I pulled into my driveway later that night. My cheeks hurt from all the grinning, but that was the last thing I cared about. She checked yes and that is all that mattered to me.

From that night on, we continued our courtship, enjoying many nights filled with wonderful meals prepared right in front of our eyes at Teppanyaki Japanese restaurant in Riverside Plaza. One night, we came across a photo booth and took a set of pictures. This started a tradition of taking silly, fun, and kissy photos at each and every photo booth we saw any time afterwards.

I had truly fallen in love with Natalia as well as her fashionable style. I especially loved when she wore a bandana in her hair, her Chucks, and a cardigan sweater, or one of her stylish old man button-up shirts she purchased from the local thrift store. Amir and I joked that she shopped at the "dead man" store.

But what I really appreciated about her, was that when she walked into a room, whether showing up at a house party or for work, she instantly lit up the entire place. She had a manner about her that was very calming, especially in stressful situations.

She wasn't perfect of course, and she was hardly ever on time for our dates and we joked that she was always, "passing Adams," which is a local street here. "I'm passing Adams" texts gave me an idea of her ETA, as well as a good laugh.

Even though she was always running late, her smile, kindness, and the comfort she brought to others, always made her worth the wait. She even turned out to be a great poker player!

It was so refreshing to be dating a girl that I loved being around, and I loved the fact that my friends immediately took to her. They

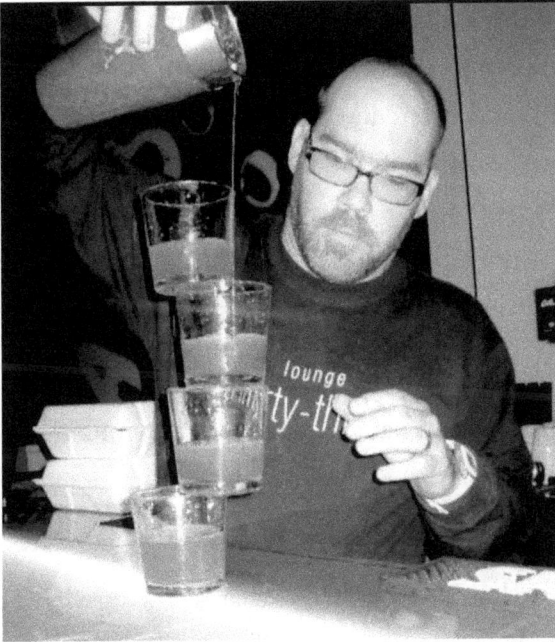

Bartending at Lounge 33

too, could tell she was a different kind of girl, with a truly authentic nature and that was a beautiful thing. I had really struck gold and I was so grateful I had found this great woman as well as her loving and generous family.

That fateful December night when all I had planned on was checking out the holiday lights downtown, led to so much more. Three years later, after many nights full of tacos and beers, movie nights and great conversations, I was elated to get Flo and Amir's blessing at her cousin's wedding. After I proposed to her in a photo booth, I followed up that incredible night by surprising her with a party full of all of our closest friends to celebrate at Lounge 33, the new bar I was working at.

As we started planning the wedding, I jumped right in to help. I even helped find the yellow bridesmaids dresses and took part in a Sexy Legs contest to win our wedding cake cutlery. Long story!

But in the midst of all the excitement of planning that special day, I got a phone call that my biological Dad was in the hospital. Both Natalia and I were in the middle of our bartending shifts, but as soon as we heard, we dropped everything and got on the road. We drove almost 300 miles to the news that my Dad had cirrhosis of the liver and was not doing well at all. His unhealthy lifestyle had finally caught up with him and it was sad to see.

I walked up to his bedside and held his hand.

"Come on Dad, hang in there. I want you at my wedding in three weeks."

"I'll do my best," he replied weakly.

It was so hard to see him like that, knowing what a competitive and athletic man he once was. A former 6'1" quarterback in high school, my Dad was always full of great football stories. No matter what, dad never seemed to lose his competitive spirit, especially off of the field. He would often beat me in darts and insist on me announcing to everybody within earshot that I was beaten by him.

He also had a lighthearted side and would always say the same thing to me every time I visited him.

"Boy, am I glad you're here. Now I don't have to be the ugliest guy in the house."

I would never forget the time I visited and had just gotten my left ear pierced. This happened to be during a family reunion, so he had more of an audience than usual. I knew as soon as he saw the earring he would say something, and I was right. As soon I stepped inside, he rubbed his red beard and then grabbed my left ear.

"That's cute."

I knew that wasn't meant to be a compliment, he actually was calling me a sissy.

"I thought you said you were gonna stand up to him, Donnie."

That was my younger brother Brad egging us on. My Dad and I started slap boxing playfully until he suddenly stopped, and took off his gold watch, and put it on the kitchen counter. As soon as he turned around, I hit him with a hook to his left rib cage, which stopped his flow. He gave me a look of respect, knowing that for once, I was the victor. This time around he had to announce that he had been beaten. We ended up hugging it out and agreed not to let things get that far anymore, as I had broken a rib of his.

That was the night he taught me to stand up for myself. Little did I know, it would be a lesson that would serve me for a lifetime.

My dad wasn't perfect and had not always been a constant presence in my life. I only saw him a few weekends a year when he came to pick up me and my two brothers, Tom and Brad. My older sister Lisa went to live with him when she became a teen, but we all remained close. Getting to his house was a respite many times, especially because it gave me a break from our Mom whose behavior could often be unpredictable due to her being bi-polar. Despite this, she was still loving and supportive, despite her own challenges, and always showed up for my baseball games.

Dad and I had a unique bond because of our mutual love for baseball and the fact that I was more drawn to sports than my other siblings.

As I recounted all of the memories that I had with him, I was interrupted by the announcement that visiting hours were ending. I looked at this thin shell of the man I once knew and gave him a kiss.

"Dad, I love you, and I better see you at my wedding in a few weeks."

He slowly raised his left hand as high as he could get it and gave me his customary thumbs up.

"I'll – be – there."

I'm sure he thought he would, but his body gave out on him.

We arrived the following day to see my Aunt Penny, a retired nurse, at his bedside with a look on her face that was telling. Unlike before, Dad now had a bunch of tubes and wires coming out of his nose and mouth.

"I love you, Dad."

Aunt Penny left the room to speak to the doctor and shortly afterwards, that same doctor unplugged the machine.

"I think that was his last breath."

My siblings stood around his bed, holding hands, and just like that, he was gone. No more pulse, no more jokes, no more beers. He was gone.

Since he loved Old Spice cologne and one of my fondest memories of him was him splashing it on my face as a kid, we decided to have his ashes transferred into a bottle of his favorite scent. Natalia and I planned to give that bottle a front row seat at our wedding. It wouldn't be him, but it would be in spirit, and that's all I could ask for.

Xavier, Jeremy, Tom, and my friends Jason and Joey from my job, were my groomsmen. I took another liberty and threw myself a "man" shower by making a deal with the local family-owned liquor store in town, La Bodega. They carry a great selection, so I made a list of all of the top shelf liquor I liked and created a registry. The owner loved the idea I had come up with and I'm pretty sure some other men came along behind me to follow in the new tradition I had started.

So, I had my "man shower," and Natalia had her bridal shower. Later that day my groomsmen and I all played eighteen holes of golf and went back home to celebrate with drinks and poker.

The following day I went to Dick's Barber shop in Riverside which I had been going to since I was twelve years old. It was pretty funny because the amount of hair I now had on my head, hardly qualified for a haircut, but it was great to hang out with Dick and Larry for a while. I was such a fixture there that I even knew their mailman! We had some good times that day!

After I was all cleaned up, we picked up my black suit, and they took me home. The wedding the following day was now the only thing left to check off.

We had a great homemade cake baked by a good friend of Natalia's, and we hired our friends for photography, music, and bartending. One of them even served as our officiant for our ceremony.

Natalia's parents agreed to have the ceremony in their spacious and lush backyard. We had a catered meal for the two hundred plus guests. They all enjoyed the photo booth, the open bar, and celebrating this new milestone in our lives with us.

As I walked down towards the altar with both my Mom, and Flo Mamma, on either side, I smiled like a kid.

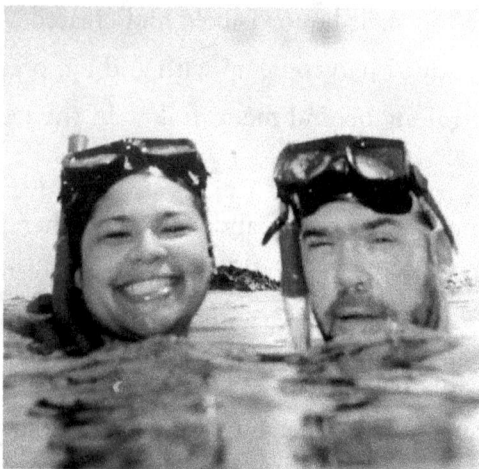

Me and Natalie 2008 – Cancun on our Honeymoon.

I couldn't wait to see Natalia!

When I heard that snare beat that starts off the song, "Invincible" by Muse, she appeared at the exact moment Muse sang:

Cause there's no one like you in the universe

I could hardly contain myself!

There she is! Oh My Holy God – this is really happening!

That beautiful brown eyed lady, who caught my eye that fateful night at The Dub, was about to say, "I do" to me!

And she did!

I kissed the bride and we walked hand in hand as Mr. & Mrs. Edison to the Rolling Stones hit, "Start Me Up." at Tom's suggestion. My once curly-haired brother, Tom, who was now bald was not only the scholar of our family, but he had also introduced me to some of my favorite music; like The Smiths and REM, so I totally trusted his judgment.

His advice was right on because the opening guitar riff of Start Me Up is so well known, and it carries a whole lot of energy. We walked by the pool holding hands and we couldn't stop smiling. The best part was when we took our first photo booth shot as a married couple.

Afterwards Flo Mamma pulled me to the side and gave me a serious look and said, " The only way out of this family is in a box."

I can't tell you what her words meant to me. The rest of the day went so great. Our guest ate, drank and danced and we had to do last call on the photo booth. Pretty funny because we didn't have to do last call on the alcohol.

We spent the night at The Mission Inn and as we were settling in, and Natalia was showering, my eyes landed on a plate of chocolate covered strawberries. In all of the excitement I had only eaten a couple of bites of dinner.

Now, here I was on my damn wedding night, the night before we were heading off to our Mexican honeymoon with low blood sugar issues. In a panic, I scarfed down most of the strawberries leaving only two for Natalia.

That was not the first time I had done something like that. It was just one of the bad habits I had developed in my childhood that I never grew out of....

CHAPTER 3

Coral Tree

After getting married, Natalia and I stayed in a large Spanish style apartment in downtown Riverside. Since both of us bartended and made pretty good money, we had the ability to save up to buy a new home. Eventually we found a cute little yellow single-story house on a cul-de-sac.

Since the house was on a quiet dead-end street, it easily passed Amir's safety check for location, which was important to both of us, but especially for him. Amir may have been just a little overprotective of Natalia, so it eased my mind to have her in a place he felt good about. In addition, it was also centrally located, within a mile of the main freeway and less than a mile from the grocery store.

Although we loved the house, we still wanted to make some changes to make it more to our liking.

There was a giant tree that stood tall directly in front of the picture windows in the front of the house. It provided much needed shade in this hot summer city, but the backyard needed the most attention. There was a cement slab back there that could fit a patio table and barbeque grill, but we had another idea.

I was not Mr. DIY by any means, but I was going to give my best shot at building a fire pit in our bare looking back yard. We were still young and were more interested in hosting friends outside than inside the house.

It was in the early stages of starting to build the fire pit that everything changed.

CHAPTER 4

Please Pull Over

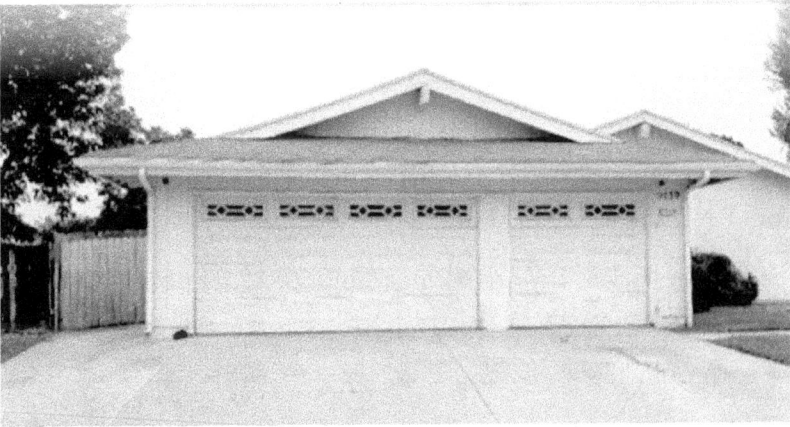

Our House 2008

It was 1980, I sat sandwiched between my younger brother Bradley on my left and my older brother Tommy on my right, in the back seat of our father's brand new 1980 maroon Datsun 200sx, his mid-life crisis purchase.

We were listening to the demo because the single by the group Soft Cell would not hit record stores until the following year. Dad brought this new cassette tape back from Germany while he was there on a business trip, and that was the only song we would hear on that two-hour drive from Canoga Park. Since this was the early eighties, there weren't a lot of alternative ways to listen to music in a car. Your only options were the radio, an eight track, or a cassette tape.

Dad would usually stop at the Topanga exit at the QuikTrip. He would buy soft drinks and snacks for us kids while making sure to fill his 7-Up bottle with the cheapest mini bottle of vodka the market sold.

Dad had a husky build and his red beard made him stand out in a crowd. He was a proud Irishman, and his beard was proof.

"Dad, I gotta pee."

I had another reason for not wanting to hear that damn song for a seventh time. I was only seven years old, but I knew I couldn't hold it in two more hours. We were still in the valley, pretty far away from Riverside where my Mom lived.

So, he locked my other three siblings in the car (this was allowed in the eighties) and walked me up to the counter to request the bathroom keys.

It was more than obvious to us, he just wanted to get us back home to our mother so he could hit the bottle with zero regard. We were still too young to comprehend the fact that our dad was drinking and driving, much less the particular dangers it held. It wasn't until I finished my RC Cola, and still had an extremely parched mouth ten minutes later, that I made a discovery.

Feeling severely thirsty, I inadvertently reached for his Diet 7-Up that was sitting in the center console. I took a sip of a very bitter liquid.

"What the heck is this?"

My eyes nearly ejected out of my face at the taste of that straight crap vodka. With my Dad's level of alcoholism, he didn't need to mix his vodka with anything. It was camouflaged by the white Diet 7-Up label so the CHP officers wouldn't bother him, but it definitely didn't have one drop of soda inside. Never mind the fact four of his own flesh and blood were depending on him to get us home to our mother alive and well.

After about five more runs of "Tainted Love," we almost had no choice but to sing along with the track:

> *Sometimes I feel I've got to run away,*
> *I've got to get away from the pain*
> *that you drive into the heart of me*

The good thing about it was the singing helped distract us from the fact it was such a long drive.

> *The love we share seems to go nowhere*
> *and I've lost my light*
> *for I toss and turn I can't sleep at night*

We memorized that part, too.

"Dad, can you please pull over again so I can pee?"

"Again? We just stopped five miles ago," he sighed. Then, "There's a gas station at the next off ramp."

Dad took the exit off the 101 at Lankershim Boulevard and pulled into the Shell station.

"Donnie let's go. The rest of you just stay quiet, and we'll be right back."

In the meantime, Tommy, Bradley, and Lisa were probably trying to conjure up how to throw that damn Soft Cell tape out of the window. They must have lost the nerve, because we made it back in a flash and the tape hadn't moved. We jumped back on the 101, and again, I got that feeling.

"Dad, is there a gas station coming up soon? I have to pee, again."

He looked at me with a stranger look than before, and without a word pulled over at the next exit.

"Okay kids, you know the drill, let's go Donnie."

As I walked into yet another public bathroom, I started to feel bad. *I only drank one RC Cola a long time ago. But I had to keep asking Dad to pull over a bunch of times!* I was also surprised he wasn't super upset with me, which made it even more confusing.

"What's wrong with me?"

"I think I may know, but it's really hard to explain. Ask your mother about it when we get there."

Two hours later we finally pulled into the driveway on Sunnyside Drive to the house Dad still legally owned half of. While on the porch, Mom attentively listened to my Dad explain why she should take me to the doctor as soon as she could.

She was wearing her traditional at home wear, which was one of any number of robes with floral patterns, accompanied by hard soled sandals that clunked across the concrete porch. Her gray hair, wrinkles and frail figure often had people assuming she was older than she really was. Her decades of smoking gave her a distinguished rasp in her voice as well as an unmistakable cough that would erupt from her lungs periodically. All four of us kids would often beg and plead with her to quit smoking. We may have just been kids, but we knew it wasn't good for her.

We all had looks of amazement on our faces when the four of us walked inside the house. We spread out on the matching couch and loveseat with the hideous brown floral print. We just couldn't believe how well our recently divorced parents were getting along. We were used to the octave level being through the roof so to speak. Seeing both of our parents keeping their cool was not normal and the look of concern on their faces during their conversation was the reason why. We were children who didn't understand the seriousness of the numerous restroom breaks.

***

The next day I was sitting in class when all of the sudden my Mom arrived and pulled me out of class. Apparently, that was the only time we could get into see Dr. Lynaweaver, my pediatrician. I was excited to get out of class and thought it made me really special. I grinned the whole time I packed up my book bag, feeling my classmates' eyes on me. I just knew they were jealous of me.

That feeling began to dissipate as I walked into that cold doctor's office holding my Mom's hand. We both sat down on the ugly brown chairs that were provided, and I finally got up the guts to ask the burning question.

"Why are we here Mommy? What's wrong with me?"

Mom had a look on her face that told a story that a seven-year-old could not pick up on.

"I don't know."

To this day I think she did but just was afraid to say it. She was thirty-seven and didn't just fall off the turnip truck.

A little while later a nurse in a stark white uniform walked in and asked me to go pee in the cup she handed to me. There was no fancy revolving mini door to put the pee sample in, so I just carried it out and handed it to the nurse. Then I rejoined my Mom in the stale, cold room.

"Well, I am pretty certain of your son Donnie's diagnosis."

Dr. Lynaweaver, a tall skinny pale white man with a terrible comb-over, was seated in his comfy chair with wheels. He rolled directly in front of us and looked Mom straight in the eyes.

"Please don't tell me it's what I think it is."

"It seems like just yesterday that Donnie was born right here in this hospital. But today," Dr. Lynaweaver composed himself, "I'm sorry to tell you that Donnie has Diabetes."

I had never heard that term before, but when my Mom started crying, that told me that whatever this Diabetes was, it was a bad thing. I laid my head on her shoulder and cried right along with her as she rubbed my head.

"You'll be okay. We'll get through this."

The way she rubbed my head felt good, but I still had no idea what "this" was.

Before I knew it, I was admitted into Riverside Community Hospital, which was an elevator ride and a few floors up away. The nurses wasted no time in training me on how to draw insulin into a syringe, which was followed by me practicing how to pinch and inject the contents of the syringe into a sponge. I was trying to be the best insulin injector into a sponge that those nurses had ever seen. I had no idea I was being prepared for a life-long routine, and it didn't even occur to me to be afraid.

It's possible that I inherently knew that complaining about what I had to do was not going to change my circumstance. I just focused on learning how to draw that insulin out of those tiny insulin bottles and jabbing my leg or stomach with the tiniest of needles. I honestly couldn't really feel them so that probably helped aid my ignorance about the severity of the situation. My Mom probably saw my focus as my superpower, but again I thought it was a game. As an athlete at an early age, I just wanted to play my best.

I was a pretty tough kid and at that point I'd been in the hospital for stitches at least five times for sports injuries, so needles were no biggie to me. If only I had kept this focus on my health, I would have a very different life right now and you wouldn't be reading this book. As a tough kid I would have gotten a 10 on a scale of 1 to 10, but as I grew older, my health would have been ranked a 0 after my diagnosis.

After about four days in the hospital, when they felt I was fully trained on drawing and injecting insulin, and how much starch and protein I should eat with each meal, I was sent home. But things would never be the same.

Unlike before, I could no longer just eat what I wanted, when I wanted. If I did, I would feel crazy, there was a new still-hard-to-describe feeling of being shaky, sweaty, confused, and a bunch of other adjectives. This would happen when my glucose level got too low, that when others saw me in this state, they tried their darndest to shove chocolate or orange juice down my throat.

This is a damn tricky disease, and at seven years old it was hard for me to comprehend the fact that it was bad to eat too much sugar and bad to not have enough. It was also bad to allow my glucose level to get too low. Since having low blood sugar gave me a feeling like I was in the Twilight Zone, nothing made sense, especially when I was at my Dad's for the weekend. When I visited him, I would often find myself somewhat conscious, until the sugar I was fed started kicking in and my full consciousness would eventually return.

One of my most vivid memories of that year, was in my Dad's apartment in the Canoga Park section of Los Angeles. At the time I was in a diabetic coma and had finally started coming to. My Dad was trying to spoon-feed me sugar, and I began to urinate in my blue Batman Underoos with the bright yellow waistband. I didn't have much awareness at that moment. If I did, I would have been embarrassed to be pissing on myself in front of him, my two brothers, and sister.

But thankfully what I remember most about that day was not the puddle of piss on that atrocious brown carpet, but the genuine concern and unconditional love that my siblings and Dad showed me.

PLEASE PULL OVER

****

I loved chocolate milk as a child and it could have very easily been the death of me...

"Yippee!"

Friday was finally here! In the eighties, certain days were designated for "special" lunch items, and Fridays were for chocolate milk. When the twelve-noon school bell rang, my fellow snot nosed first grade peers and I were forced to walk in a single file line. We were supposed to line up on the painted line on the concrete path to the cafeteria, but Scotty G refused. Scotty always seemed to cause a little ruckus, and this would usually be followed by Bernadette, the lunch marshal, blowing her whistle. She always walked at an agonizing snail's pace, as her eyes pierced through the crowd of little rascals just itching to open their carton of Swiss dairy chocolate milk. Her stare alone seemed to be enough to get those kids back into a straight line.

Everything about the way things were going was familiar, except this was the first Friday I felt like an outsider.

"Donnie, Oh Donnie boy can't have chocolate milk."

I was on my way to give the cashier my lunch number. A lunch number was for a student like me who was too poor to afford to buy lunch. I tried best not to get in line next to that cutie pie Dawn, hoping she didn't know my family's economic status. It would be hard not to, based on my holey Toughskins and worn-down sneakers, but I still thought I might have a shot. I just knew I didn't want her to hear the lunch lady call out my number and see me get the ticket, because then she would surely know how poor I really was. Thankfully, she wasn't part of Scotty's crew engaged in that chant which only quieted when Bernadette stared them down.

"Donnie can't have chocolate milk because he's got a disease."

I knew what I was supposed to do but...

As silly as that may seem, like most first graders, I just wanted to fit in and for people to like me. *Those little punks weren't going to do that to me*! I slid my bright orange tray down the stainless-steel counter with my soggy green beans and boxed mashed potatoes which were slopped on the off-white and overly used plastic plate. I walked in front of the lunch lady who held the tray with the white and chocolate milks. The white milk was still covered in plastic wrap. The peer pressure and embarrassment I knew I would feel would not allow me to cave in to doing what I knew I was supposed to.

"Chocolate, please."

I looked over my right shoulder out of the habit of watching out for my mother who was always trying to make sure I did the right thing, especially in regard to my diet. I felt like I had to do something to shut those punks up. When I walked away with the chocolate milk, I knew I had a victory because now my lunch tray looked just like theirs, so they would have nothing to say.

This became my Friday routine complete with the look over my right shoulder for mother. I knew deep down I should not be drinking that damn chocolate milk. *But it was so good though!* I also didn't have to put up with those punks. Problem solved, right? Now that's where my naiveté hit its pinnacle.

Since I kept getting away with it, I eventually got even more daring and by the time I got to middle school, the routine was firmly set in place. I would walk up to the snack bar and order chocolate milk *and* mini powdered donuts.

How are these few little donuts gonna hurt me?

34

The doctors, as well as my Mom would often say things like, "Take care of your diabetes," or "You don't want to go blind or lose a limb, do you?"

The answer was an obvious no, but I had embraced a belief that kept me going.

None of that would ever happen to me!

I would not consider myself a pathological liar in the slightest, but it was easiest to lie to my dad, especially since I saw him less than my mom. Whenever he asked me how I was doing with taking care of my diabetes, I had the perfect answer rehearsed for him.

"Good, just fine." I could deliver this lie without the slightest stutter every single time. I always made sure to use different variations of the response each time so it wouldn'tsound as scripted as it was. I felt invincible, with the way I could hide it from both of my parents. I reveled in that fact that I could do whatever I wanted to when they weren't looking, so I could enjoy my young life.

Those years of disobedience from elementary to middle school, displayed my blatant disregard for this fucking disease called diabetes. But by the time I got to high school, I took it to an even higher level.

After the fourth period bell would sound, me, Xavier and the other guys would meet at the lockers and throw our books in. With our upcoming trip a whole lot lighter, we burst through the school doors, and made our way to the chain linked fence that separated our school from the Amber Gate Apartments.

Once we climbed the ten foot fence to get to cross from the school side, we threw our legs over, and rested a moment while our balls got smashed by the crossbar at the top of the fence. After each of us reached the other side, we ran like a pack of starving wolves until we reached a seven foot high cinder block wall on the other side where a paradise of fast food awaited us.

We had our choice of Del Taco (AKA "Club Del"), or Yum Yum Donuts. At least a couple of days a week we would hit up the Yum Yum where the five of us would polish off a dozen of those glazed circles of deliciousness. I always made sure that two of the twelve always had my name on them.

I knew I was doing just fine since my friends didn't say anything and my parents were clueless. I figured that since nobody that gave a shit knew, it was no big deal.

Club Del was the best because it was the cheapest of them all, especially because the five of us could share a Dr. Pepper fountain drink. Not wanting to be the odd man out, I would just guzzle it down like the rest of them.

We had a saying between us, "You finish, you fill."

The guy who took the last drink had to go refill the cup, and that wasn't the worst of it. We'd top it off with a smoke. This was before the indoor smoking restrictions of the late eighties. Since my buddies smoked cigarettes, so did I.

It was nothing to have a sleepover at one of the guys' houses with no parents around and polish off a twelve pack of Budweiser and some smokes. I did this over and over again even though I'd always end up paying for my actions at midnight when I was in the bathroom hovering over the toilet.

Why the hell did I do that?

I had no idea and didn't bother to answer because the routine was such a part of my life. It got to the point where I got so used to it, that I didn't get sick anymore.

The motto, *"If nobody made me feel bad for my behavior despite having a serious disease, what was the harm?"* Worked for me for years.

So, with my glazed donut lunches, after-meal cigarettes, and beer filled weekends I had it made. The fact that I kept fooling my Mom made it seem like I was foolproof. Though to be honest, sometimes I felt like she had just given up, and stopped trying to be the authority of the household. Most likely if I felt this way it was due to her continuing mental health and financial struggles since my Dad was often late with child support. I still hated it when she bothered me about taking care of myself but in retrospect, I appreciate that she kept trying.

The sad truth is, that I got so used to doing whatever the hell I wanted, that many people had no idea I was a diabetic.

In reality, with a disease like diabetes, everyone I was ever around should have not just known but should have had some understanding of what to do if I ever went into a low blood sugar episode. If that would have happened, and they didn't know what to do, it would not have been a good situation.

Fortunately for them and me, that never happened. It is super ironic that my awful diet and lifestyle actually prevented me from having low blood sugar. My friends were spared from seeing an episode, and being the careless teenager I was, I never thought it would catch up with me.

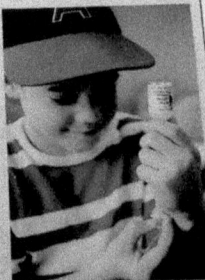

PROMOTING
Communi
RIVERSIDE COMMUNIT
CONTINUING EDUCATI

DONNY EDISON
is a 7-year old diabetic
who was admitted last
November with juve-
nile diabetes. His love
for baseball is evident
by his picture.

Learning the tricks of the
trade at 7 years old in
1980.

A few years after graduating from high school, I had a few conversations with some of my closest friends about my behavior. They
all shared the same philosophy about my unhealthy lifestyle. Although they knew I wasn't supposed to be having lots of sugar, they
weren't going to tell me what to do. We were all young and dumb
and I don't fault them, because to tell you the truth it was my respon-
sibility, not theirs.

CHAPTER 5

Ballard

Wow, those were some wild dreams last night...

I realized none of it was a dream when I woke up in my hospital bed after my first night at Ballard rehabilitation hospital. I felt lucky that I had the bed by the window so I could see the sun shining in. I looked to my left at the curtain that separated me from my roommate, instantly feeling bad that he wasn't able

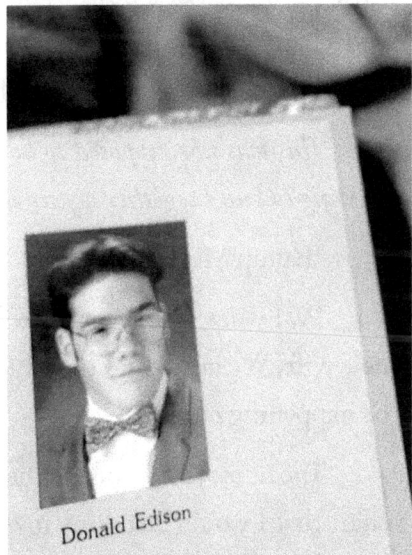

Donald Edison

Senior Photo, 1991

to see the sun. After checking out the rest of the room I looked down at myself, and as sure as I was breathing, I saw something that didn't seem right.

I had to be seeing things!

The doctor did say that my vision might be impaired so that had to be it.

"Why are you wearing a diaper?"

Natalia's question confirmed my eyes were not playing tricks on me.

"Oh! It is a diaper? I wasn't sure, but now that I know, I am extremely embarrassed."

"It's not a big deal. I'll ask the nurse to put your boxers on."

To my relief, she headed out to the nurse's station and a few moments later, the kind nurse came in and put my boxers on. She then proceeded to get me into the chair next to the bed for my breakfast which consisted of a bowl of plain cheerios, a piece of wheat bread, and a banana. Natalia sat and watched me, and I could only imagine what thoughts were going on in her head.

This was not supposed to be part of the new life we had only just starting to build together a year earlier!

"Eat up Mr. Edison."

"Why am I here? It's not fair. I'm only thirty-six. This is my new wife. We just bought our house a few weeks ago. This shouldn't be happening to me."

The nurse just shook her head and transferred me to the wheelchair that I would be taking my shower on.

"Just be glad you didn't wait any longer. You could have been a goner."

I was so scared. It couldn't believe how much I wasn't able to do on my own! The next thing I knew I was naked on a wheelchair in the shower with a nurse watching over me. *Talk about having all my pride thrown out of the window!* I felt completely helpless at that moment. Once I was all cleaned up, the nurse got me dressed, and put on my socks, my boxers, and a pair of sweatpants Natalia brought.

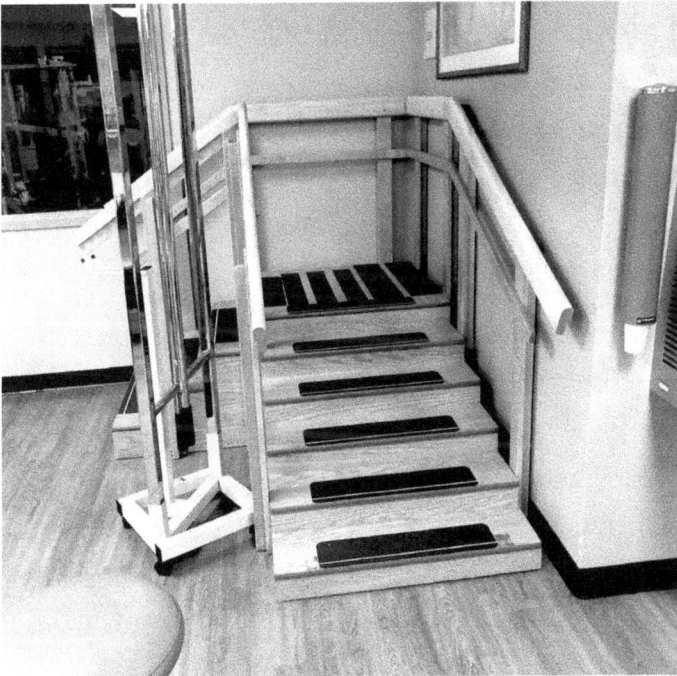

The **Huge** Staircase

A sweet young woman with smiling eyes approached me.

"Hi! I'm your physical therapist, Amy."

Amy got me in my wheelchair and pushed me towards the exit.

"Work hard, Donnie."

Natalia gave me a kiss and Amy and I headed to the gym for physical therapy.

"I can't believe this happened to me," is all I could say as we headed to the entrance of the therapy gym. When we got there, the first thing I saw was the mock staircase.

"So, Amy, when do I get to walk up those stairs?"

She smirked. "Donnie, you can't even stand up by yourself yet, but that's a great goal."

What the hell am I going to do? Life was going so well, Natalia and I were both making pretty good money, we took trips when we wanted, and now I needed someone to stand in the bathroom with me while I'm sitting on the can? I have to open my mouth after I swallow a bite of food to make sure I don't choke. Holy shit! It was all taken from me just like that! All gone!

I made eye contact with a few more patients before my first workout session, and soon realized we all had the same sad story about how this wasn't fair. It wasn't doing me any good, but I did it anyway. Amy laid me down on the raised padded mat and helped me stretch. Then she stood me up and wrapped a safety belt around my waist as I attempted to walk around the mat which was about thirty feet in total distance. After only one lap, I was already tired. *What the hell?*

"I can't be tired already."

"That's very normal, Donnie. Don't beat yourself up about it. We will keep working for the next few weeks and you'll start to see improvements. You'll see."

I wanted to believe her, but I must admit I wasn't so sure. I was scared because I couldn't just do what I wanted like I was used to. I was also afraid that other people would see me fall. I still viewed myself as a healthy young man, but in reality, I had lost 95% of the right hemisphere of my brain, and young is an extremely relative term.

I went ahead and walked around the mat a few more times and decided to save my complaining for after I finished.

"Donnie, stop talking so you can concentrate better."

I took Amy's cue and figured if I walked really slowly, I could save my complaining for when I could tell a fresh pair of ears. Before she took me to the cafeteria for lunch, I had complained to about twenty different people.

After lunch, Amy drove me over to Mike's office for more speech therapy. Mike needed to check my cognitive function again. He asked me what my favorite card game was.

"Texas Hold' em is my favorite."

He proceeded to pull a deck of cards out of his desk drawer and we used paper clips as our money.

"What makes you a good poker player?"

"I often know what cards my opponents are holding."

As Mike dealt the first hand, he mentioned that he was interested in seeing what I was talking about. After I won a bunch of his paper clips on the first hand, he studied me.

"What cards was I holding?"

"I feel like you had King 10,"

He smiled and shook his head.

"King 9. How did you do that?"

"There were a couple different things. I noticed the way you were betting, and how disappointed you looked when that queen you were looking for to make a straight, didn't come."

Even with that victory, I still found time to complain to Mike about what happened to me and how unfair it was. After about an hour of playing, my Occupational therapist Stacey came in and introduced herself.

"You'll be learning how to get dressed only using one hand."

How hard could that be?

No more than twenty minutes later, I was about in tears trying to put on my socks.

"Please let me put on my shirt."

That was a much easier task, because I could see the arm holes much better than the hole where my foot goes into a sock.

Damn my vision is scary bad!

Stacy got a couple of earfuls of complaints from me. She let me go on and on, and after a couple hours of me figuratively crying, the day was nearly over. She wheeled me to the cafeteria for dinner, and I got myself back in complaint mode.

When my daily grilled cheese and tomato soup showed up, I actually found myself a smile. My kind of comfort food, even though I still had to open my mouth after each swallow, to make sure I didn't choke. I picked up my bowl of soup to drink the final drop and complained because I was hoping to get something sweet with dinner. The nurse that was monitoring my swallows reminded me to look at the left side of the plate, *Bam, there it was! Applesauce*!

"Because of your blindness on your left peripheral, the person who sets your food tray down puts the dessert on your left to ensure that you practice scanning to see everything."

After that long day of therapy from morning to night, I was very tired. After dinner I sat and watched a little baseball, and Stacy wheeled me to my room for bed. I knew I was doing better because I only complained once on the way there. As we entered my room, I decided that I needed to have a little conversation with myself.

Donnie, do you feel any better about your new situation to-night than you did earlier today?"

"No, I don't!

"Ok well if you want to get through this, you're going to have to start being more positive, and work harder than you have ever worked, period."

It was in that moment that I reasoned with myself that though I most certainly didn't choose to have a stroke, I sure did have a choice in how I responded to it.

That much I could figure out with only a half of a brain. This philosophy made a lot of sense. I could have continued to have a sad face and complained every day, all day. I absolutely could! But I honestly wasn't so sure that would help me get through this. As an athlete, I knew that hard work and a positive attitude would give me a better shot at winning this rehabilitation game.

It was totally up to me!

That was the best conversation I had that entire day; I could no longer allow myself to go down that path of complaining. My rationale told me that working hard was the better option. In the case of playing to win, it would also be a heck of a lot more fun!

CHAPTER 6

Fridays

In 1992, I got a job waiting tables at Johnny Rockets, and after a few months of making an average of about sixty bucks a shift, and still living at home at age nineteen, I upgraded my 1967 baby blue Volkswagen Beetle that my Uncle Bill had given me. I was more than happy to say goodbye to those rusted out floorboards which caused the inside of the car to fill up with water whenever it rained.

Upgrading to my brand-new, navy blue Toyota, pick-up felt great. With a $167.00 a month car payment, a new waitress girlfriend, and new job, I was excited about how things were going.

The next morning the news that followed my Mom's usual morning knock changed my mood.

"Johnny Rockets is closed Donnie. The owner emptied it out and closed it down."

After she left, I realized I had to act fast.

Oh shit! How was I going to make my car payment?

My heart returned to my chest as I remembered my wisdom in keeping three months' worth of payments in the top drawer of my dresser. Even at that age, I knew that most things were not a guarantee. I had learned this lesson early on.

When I was eleven, I was the shortstop on the all-star little league team , and during a practice one early summer evening, the infielders were practicing fielding ground balls. Every time I had to move laterally to ground the ball to my left or right, I would slide as soon as I planted my feet. My coach finally called me over and asked to look at the bottom of my cleats, noticing there was zero traction on them.

"Can your Mom get you a new pair?"

Ashamed and embarrassed, I shook my head back and forth.

"She can't afford to."

At the end of that week, on a beautiful summer night under the lights, I approached the field as usual inhaling the smell of the fresh cut grass that I loved. My coach called me over for a team meeting. In front of everybody, he handed me a shoe-box with a brand new pair of cleats. The parents of all of my teammates had chipped in to buy them. I appreciated their kindness but still had mixed feelings. As much as I appreciated their generosity, I felt shame. But I turned it around and a new philosophy was implanted inside of me.

Just because my mom was poor didn't mean I had to be.

I learned in the moment that if I ever wanted anything, I was going to have to work for it. It was my first lesson in financial independence, and I had no idea of how important this lesson would end up being for me.

It was with this understanding that I began working by the age of fifteen, doing anything from dressing up like a clown and twirling a sign for a new tract home development, to working in a liquor store as a high school senior. That job was short-lived after a botched armed-robbery attempt, but that didn't stop me from always having a job from that point on.

By the time I was nineteen, I had plenty of work experience, so finding a new job was just going to come down to who was hiring. And even though my car payment wasn't a lot of money to me, I knew that I couldn't depend on my mom to help me.

I knew a lot of people in my hometown of Riverside, so I got out on the very day I found out I'd no longer have my waiter job. I asked everyone I knew who was working if their job was hiring.

I filled out applications everywhere I could including TGI Fridays. I got a call the following week for an interview. For the first time, the interview experience felt intimidating. A series of interviews was to follow but when I didn't get a call after the first, I called to follow up.

"Hi Emelia, this is Donnie Edison. I just wanted to know if I was going to get a second interview."

"Oh! Rosie didn't call you?

"Uh – no."

"Okay. Well can you come in on Thursday afternoon then?

"Sure thing, Emelia, thank you."

My follow up paid off! That interview led to my working at Fridays as a waiter and eventually bartender for over thirteen years. Had I not gotten embarrassed on that baseball field as a kid, I might not have had the tenacity to get that second interview so quickly.

Fridays was a lot busier and more expensive than Johnny Rockets, so I was now making eighty to one hundred bucks a shift in tips. What didn't change was my eating or drinking habits. Friday nights after work, my fellow co-workers and I would sit in the parking lot and talk over a few beers and unwind which became part of my new routine.

A year later when I turned twenty, I felt the need for greater freedom that I could not get living in my mother's house. So, I asked Tim and Thad if they would be interested in being roommates. They said yes, and to make a long story short, we found a place in Canyon Crest. It was a three bedroom for only $775.00 in a decent neighborhood.

The three of us being bachelors, got excited thinking about our own place, and parties with pretty girls. I loved the idea of having my own bathroom and told them I'd pay twenty-five extra to take the loft on top, and the guys agreed.

Our credit was decent, and we were each making roughly the same amount of money, so we were easily approved. Of course, we all celebrated with a beer even though I was a year shy of twenty-one. At that point, I had been going out once a week with my friends for a beer. But now that I lived with guys who were drinking age, this number was going to increase.

Drinking in excess is not a good habit for anyone, but for a diabetic it is a much more serious problem. But I continued to live in a crazy way of thinking, always reasoning that as long as I had all of my limbs, fingers, and my sight, that I was okay. My denial continued to tell me so.

We moved in a month before my twenty-first birthday, and by that time our place was known for being well-stocked with bottles of liquor, ice chests of beer, and special drink shots were written on a piece of cardboard as a drink menu.

I did admit to myself that the shots tasted like shit, but they had funny names and helped get people drunk, so I just got used to it. There were about a handful of guests that were under the age of twenty-one, so when the cops showed up, I went into action. I had a great talent for keeping my body from swaying and my speech from slurring.

"Is everyone here over the age of twenty-one?"

"Yes, Officer."

"Make sure it stays that way if you don't want to see us again."

"Yes Sir."

Once the officer pulled off, I addressed the party.

"If any of you are too drunk to drive at 3 a.m. then you can sleep over. If you are not, then you need to go."

3 a.m. was the best time to shut everything down. We were pretty loud and didn't want to make the neighbors mad again.

This was the lifestyle I didn't give a second thought to. But my body would pay for it later.

CHAPTER 7

A New Attitude and A New Friend

When Natalia showed up on day two after my stroke, it was lunch-time. I was not able to sit in my room alone because of the color of my pink wristband. Every patient admitted had a wristband that correlated with their abilities, and pink meant I could not, under any circumstances, be left alone. By the time Natalia arrived, I was sitting in my wheelchair in the hallway across from the nurse's station alongside the other "pinkies", who all ranged in age, gender, and ethnicity.

"What are you doing out here in the hall?"

"Just hanging out with my cronies." I joked.

She shook her head at me, laughed, and shook her head again. She knew me so well.

On day two of rehab, I had to swallow my pride and let the nurse help me get dressed. It was hard for me to accept that I, a thirty-six-year-old man, needed someone else to help me get my boxer shorts, socks, t-shirt, and shoes on.

I was sure my frustration could be seen right there on my face for everyone to see.

I have been doing this stuff all my life!

But something deep inside of me decided to change my mindset that morning, thanks to the conversation I had with myself. I got up at seven a.m. for breakfast, showered, dried off to the best of my ability and promised myself that I would do all of these things again for myself without anyone's help. This attitude is probably why I am still here today.

Don't get me wrong, my frustration wasn't going to just automatically disappear. By the time I'd gotten to the gym for my physical therapy and spoke to the breakfast lady, my nurses and physical therapist did not hear me complain one time. I knew that my life *seemed* to be upside down, but I was determined to reverse that. I did everything that was asked of me, so if my therapist asked me to do fifteen leg lifts, they did not hear me complain – I did twenty.

Come on Donnie just one more! You can do it!

Even after a full day of therapy mixed in with a lunch break, I kept my attitude even though I wasn't moving too well. I also made sure to encourage other patients in the gym.

The biggest complaint I had was the day I went to speech therapy and my therapist Mike didn't play poker like we usually did. Instead, he had me work on some cognitive exercises. He then told me a color, a two-digit number, and a food item then we would have a conversation for about thirty seconds. After that he would immediately ask me to repeat the two-digit number he gave me.

I was optimistic because Mike gave an A grade and told me my memory didn't seem to be too affected from the stroke. I just added it to my list of things to be grateful for. Later that evening in the cafeteria for dinner, I asked the nurse to please park me at the table in front of the sixty inch TV so I could see the ballgame. Along with the delicious grilled cheese sandwich and tomato soup, I was pretty good. My soup was a little cold, and though I knew it wasn't much to complain about in the grand scheme of things, I asked DD to warm it up for me.

As I watched him take it over to the microwave about ten steps away, I didn't focus on the fact that I couldn't physically do the same yet. I thanked him, shook his hand, and continued watching the game. He was a real nice guy and had heard enough of my complaints the day before. But I was determined to make sure he wouldn't ever hear them again.

After dinner, DD wheeled me to my room for bed. As I settled in, I saw that my roommate was an older African American man that reminded me a lot of Morgan Freeman. I was still pretty shy, so I didn't speak to him right away. But after about twenty minutes of talking myself into it, I decided to start a conversation.

"Hello Sir, what's your name?"

He took a breath and smiled.

"I'm Pete, Pete Pederson, and what's your name?" he asked in a raspy voice.

"I'm Donnie Edison. So, Pete, do you happen to like baseball?"

"Oh yes, I love baseball. I actually played pro as a matter of fact," he proudly stated.

"Oh wow, what organization did you play for?"

"I played triple A for the Detroit Tigers."

"We're going to be good friends Pete! Guess who my uncle was?

"Who?"

Sparky Anderson."

"Are you kidding me?"

My day was getting even better! What were the chances my new roommate not only loves my favorite sport, but he was even a minor league right fielder for the same team my uncle managed from 1979-1995!

The reason I was such a baseball aficionado came from my mom who was Sparky's sister. She used to shag baseballs for him when she was growing up. (for non-baseball people, this means chasing the balls) My Uncle Sparky was one of the best baseball managers in the game. He managed the National League's Cincinnati Reds to the 1975 and 1976 championships, and then added a third title in 1984 with the Detroit Tigers of the American League. I didn't know him super well beyond his visits to Los Angeles to sign autographs, but his legacy is something I am definitely proud of.

So, baseball was pretty much in my blood from birth.

I still couldn't believe that of all the rooms in that hospital, I got to room with a cool older man who I could talk baseball with! From that night on until his release, Pete and I would talk in the dark. We couldn't see each other much because of the divider curtain. He would often sneak out of his bed and I teased him and called him, "Spiderman." Though he was frailer than me, he always beat me to the cafeteria every evening.

"Hey! Donnie Baseball!"

After he called out to me, I'd get my plate and we would proceed to chat about that weeks' game. We really had some good times and the fact that the two of us, of all people ended up in the same room, somehow let me know everything was going to be okay.

Our conversations would have gone on for hours if it wasn't for the fact that he was constantly pressing the nurse button for a new bedpan.

In the daytime his wife Nadia, who had great love for her husband, would visit and make sure he was well cared for. They had married late in life and neither one had kids, but they sure did love each other.

"I am so glad Pete met you." She would tell me in her European accented voice. Behind closed doors she would add, "You are so good for each other. It's been so hard for him."

I agreed and promised to stay in touch with them when I left Ballard. I knew his recovery would be more difficult since he was significantly older than I was. I used this fact as even more motivation for myself. *I really had no excuse!*

I know I was on a mission to stay positive and work my butt off, and I honestly felt much better about my situation especially compared to Pete. I kept reminding myself that my progress was possible if I just kept my mind right. This wasn't easy, but I was glad to have a friend here. I imagined us pushing each other to hit our goals.

I couldn't wait to walk again!

Most people take being able to walk for granted. But if they woke up tomorrow and couldn't, it is only then that they would understand. There are so many in our society who can't, and believe me they don't take things for granted that able-bodied people don't even think about. Unless of course, someone close to them is *diffabled*.

I don't like the word disabled. *Diffabled* just means that people have a different way of doing things. I feel disabled has such a negative connotation to it and as you may have figured out, I am a pretty positive person!

CHAPTER 8

Start the Party

I was glad that we figured out all of these strategies to keep me safe, but I still couldn't forget the way I had lived my life and how it had caught up with me especially as a young adult.

These were the days where I was glad that those days of looking over my shoulder to see if someone would report me for drinking chocolate milk were finally over. I was an adult and there was nobody to tell me what I should do with my life. Compared to now, chocolate milk seemed like holy water.

My TGI Friday's co-workers and I had a very unhealthy household, but we thought we knew everything as most twenty-somethings do.

Our kitchen had enough space between the top of the cabinets and the ceiling to fit a beer bottle, so we displayed a plethora of different brands of beer from Sam Adams, ranging from Cherry Wheat to Cream Stout, to everything in between.

We drank on the weekdays as well as the weekends. It was a way of life for us. Since we made most of our money waiting tables on the weekends, a typical weeknight with all three of us off work usually consisted of downing a couple of six packs of cold beer, along with eating microwaved burritos from Club Del or frozen ones from the local grocery store. We topped them off with hot sauce that was always in inventory in the fridge, along with milk for my bowl of Corn Flakes.

The rest of the fridge had plenty of room for what we considered the necessary items, which was even more beer. As time went on, a random bottle of liquor would usually appear on top of the refrigerator as well. This was for those nights when we felt one beer alone couldn't quite do the trick.

Our diet was probably not much different from most bachelor pads and cigarettes just added to our unhealthy lifestyle. This behavior went on for about a year until I met my match one summer night.

With a rare day shift on a Friday, one might think I would have taken it easy, but instead I tied my drunk on even tighter. My roommate Tim had invited his girlfriend over, and our other roommate Thad, invited his flavor of the week. Thad was the looker of us, so it was always a mystery which girl he would be with on any given day. I invited my current girlfriend, Cheri, over to hang out.

We ordered pizza and played drinking games until about four a.m. I had an eleven o'clock morning shift, so I set my alarm for ten. Unfortunately, I did not hear it until noon, and I shot up in bed in a panic.

This was not the typical situation where I woke up late, called in and needed to instantaneously start coming up with excuses. The day before, I had promised to cover a shift for one of my co-workers, so I needed to come up with something good. I picked up the land-line, cleared my throat and prepared my story.

"Hi Mike."

I could immediately tell from his tone that he was pissed, but I also knew that this was the first time I had been a no-show, so I had that on my side.

"Mike, my blood sugar was really low, and I woke up in a pool of sweat and confused. So, I need to eat some sugar real quick to get it back to where it should be. I'm so sorry."

"Okay."

Was he buying it? I sure hoped so.

"Do you want me to still come in or did you get someone else to cover?"

"I got it covered, but you're still getting written up."

I hung up deeply upset. *What the hell was I doing?* I knew I needed to slow my roll, but damn I had been having so much fun. But I still knew that I couldn't let this fun interfere with this good paying job that allowed me to drive a nice new truck, live on my own, and afford to treat myself.

This event made me so scared of losing my job that I stopped drinking the nights before I had to work the next morning. Although I had a very unhealthy lifestyle, I still knew that when I wanted to do something, I had to put myself in a position to do it, no matter what. From that point on, I asked to be scheduled three day shifts a week. I knew I would sacrifice financially because the tips would be smaller, but I reasoned that I also wouldn't be spending as much money on booze, so it would all even out. As long as I made enough to cover my truck payment, pay rent, eat, and take my girlfriend out once a week, I was okay with it.

My roommates didn't make any changes to their lifestyle, so I had to stay strong. My morning shifts started at eleven, so after about two weeks of listening to these guys drinking and having fun, I convinced myself that as long as I went to bed by two the night before, I'd be okay. I also made sure to eat a little something before bed to help keep my blood sugar from going too low.

I'm embarrassed to admit that although I had a blood glucose monitor all along, I never used it. There was really no excuse aside from being young and dumb, because at this point I was in full neglect mode and had no role models around me to direct me otherwise.

I just kept convincing myself I was fine, counted my fingers and kept on going. My logic was all a load of crap that I refused to see. The entire time I was allowing my condition to get worse and worse, never considering the consequences of my actions.

****

Eventually, my roommates and I decided to part ways and I moved back in with my mom. That way I could save a few hundred bucks a month and she would have some assistance with her utility bills, which she really needed. She had had her share of challenges but had always been there for me especially in regards to my playing baseball. No matter what, she had always been in the stands during my games, giving me my stats along with constructive criticism about how I had played. It was my turn to pay all that she had done for me, forward.

She was also a great example for me in discipline. Despite her terrible smoking habit, she was known around the neighborhood as, "The Walker," for her daily two-mile walks around the neighborhood. But despite me and my siblings' pleas, she never quit smoking. Even now that we were young adults, it was pretty common to see a cigarette, lit or not, hanging from her lips. We knew not to say a word about it if we were going to stay on her good side. We also knew better than to sit in "her chair", (a worn-down dark brown leather seat that she refused to throw away), when we visited.

I loved her unconditionally though I wasn't crazy about some of her choices. But she was a grown woman and at that time we both needed assistance. I was also grateful that she let me come and go as I pleased, giving me my adult freedom.

****

About six months after I moved in with mom, I found myself without a girlfriend. Soon after, I ran into Lee, a cute and stylish Japanese girl that had once gone out with an old acquaintance of mine. For once, we were both single, so I took my shot.

"Why don't we have a drink and catch up?"

The following Thursday was known as College Night at Lake Alice, the local so-called "biker bar," full of pool tables, dart boards, with liquor advertisements that lined the walls.

Even though the constant barrage of Bon Jovi and Def Leppard blaring through the static-filled speakers was beyond annoying, we enjoyed ourselves. Later on, we started swing dancing when they started playing the fifties scene music. After way too many three dollar Long Island Ice Teas, and lots of flirting, we made our way to the bar to close out the tab. Although I drove, I was pretty smashed, and Lee's car was parked in front of my Mom's house. So, we walked across University Ave in downtown Riverside to the parking lot, where my truck was parked.

How am I going to get us back safely?

"Are you okay to drive Donnie?"

"I don't know. Let's get in the car and I will see how I feel once I sit down."

I sat down. I really felt pretty out of it and whenever I looked up from my lap, I got extremely dizzy. It just seemed like everything was spinning.

"Are you too drunk?

She shrugged, "No but – I don't know how to drive stick shift."

So, my brilliant young mind decided on a totally irrational plan. I decided that I would sit in the driver's seat, press on the gas and control the clutch and shift, and she would look up and steer. Although in hindsight, this was an idiotic solution, it was the best I could come up with at the time.

Not only could we both have died that night because of my drunken stupidity, but if a police officer had seen us, I would have surely gotten arrested and charged with a DUI. At twenty-two, this was a new low for me. I was heading nowhere fast, but socializing and late nights out with pretty girls was all that I cared about.

As scary as it was, the Lake Alice incident did nothing to change my ways, especially working at one of the most happening restaurants in town. To make it worse, I actually believed that my drinking helped me become a social butterfly full of confidence. Girlfriends came and went, and there always was another standing by the bar waiting to have a drink with me. Since I had been promoted to the bartender position, liquor was even more at my disposal than ever, and my foot was still not easing off the accelerator of my dangerous lifestyle.

The last thing in the world that I was thinking about was my diabetes and never told any new friends that I had it. What made it worse was that I continued living like I didn't know I had it either.

CHAPTER 9

Final Stretch to Home Plate

Going into week three at Ballard, I was reaching all of the goals that were set by the therapists as well as myself, since day one. After an evaluation by the hospital, I was told I would be sent home at the end of the third week. Although there was a lot to celebrate, I still had quite a bit of apprehension.

"I'm worried because I feel like I still need a lot of help with most things, and there won't be nurses at home to help."

I absolutely did not want to feel like I was a burden on Natalia and didn't want to admit that I was a little scared to go home.

The job of the rehabilitation hospital is to prepare a patient to go home, and now I could walk, though I was slow as a snail. But I reminded myself that at least I could walk and get dressed on my own. I was still extremely frustrated, and almost in tears at times, but something still told me: *You can do it!*

I was heading into the final stretch of therapy which could be classified as at home living training. The final week before being discharged, I would learn how to get in and out of a shower using a shower chair by myself, and how to get up off of the ground by myself. These are basic tasks for most people, but with my loss of vision, and use of only one hand, they were quite challenging. I had to learn strategies to complete them in a new way, but despite my competitive nature, I still didn't have much confidence.

With my new "half body" getting down to the ground with only one arm and one leg, and not being able to feel or see my left limbs, was very difficult. I knew all of my limbs were there, but I couldn't feel them. This made it almost impossible to think about moving. I had to think about exactly where to put my right hand on a couch to help hoist myself up. At the same time, I had to use my right hand to move my left leg into a position that would not interfere with me getting up. With having what the therapists referred to as *left side neglect*, it wasn't second nature.

Sometimes I would entirely forget or neglect my left side as if it wasn't even there, so as one might imagine, this "simple" process of just getting upright was not so "simple." The mental strength I was now using over these past three weeks was becoming semi-autonomic in a sense. But as frustrated as I might find myself in a given situation on a daily basis, my mindset "I am going to win!" kept me from quitting.

It was still difficult to put on my socks with one hand. It was difficult to get off the ground. It was even difficult to step one foot in the shower so I could sit on a bench! This was hard because I couldn't see the end of the left side of the bench without fully rotating my head to that side. There was a lot to keep in mind all at once, all while sitting there naked in front of my nurse. Let me tell you, the mentally weak are just not cut out for this, but whether I was or not, I was determined to work at it so I would not get crushed.

At this point I had earned a blue band and could now sit in my room in my wheelchair by myself. Now I could sit and chill out in my room and watch TV if I wanted to. I was very proud of this achievement!

On my third day of new privileges, my old friend Joey stopped by with some lunch. When I reached with my right leg for the tray to get it closer to me, I suddenly found myself on the ground. That tray was obviously further away than it had appeared, and my stretch caused me to slide right out of that wheelchair. So there I was on the ground, with Joey trying to pull up one hundred and seventy five pounds of dead weight. Luckily, a nurse who was walking by saw what was going on.

After that incident, I had to wear a pink band again, but that was the least of my problems. I was sent to the hospital across the street for x-rays of my ribs. There was a bruising, but luckily nothing was broken. Either way, my final week of rehab was scrapped, and another week was added. So now I had two weeks of ICU, and rehab for four. That would now make six weeks instead of five.

That was my lesson: *Our lives change on us in an instant and we must never take anything for granted.* That is when I started to learn to be grateful for the smallest of things. Things like being able to hop in your car and drive to the market to sitting down and tying your shoes.

I never thought twice about those things before my stroke, but now all the bases were loaded, the teams were tied, and it was a whole new ball game.

I knew my perspective would be key. I no longer had the freedom to sit in my room alone, but I couldn't care less. I had to keep my eye on the prize, and that prize was getting back home to my wife and family, period.

Before I left, Natalia and I made a list of the folks we would buy a small gift for to show my appreciation for their guidance, even if it was just an ear to listen. It was our way of saying thank you.

***

The final step in my being released was that the therapists had to teach Natalia how to safely transfer me from my wheelchair to the car, and back. It was not just sling that left leg in first, sit on butt, and shut the door. Oh no, it was much more involved and deliberate:

With my back facing the inside of the car, I would sit both of my butt cheeks on the seat, then grab my left leg with my right hand and pull my left leg into the car. Then I could get my right leg in the car. Nothing was simple anymore.

I was determined to get through this, and with a smile, even though I knew it wasn't going to be easy. That was okay with me because I knew I had done this to myself. I just hated that all of this was disrupting Natalia's life of freedom and traveling.

Talk about a strong woman, boy oh boy, what an amazing soul she was to me under these tough circumstances. I had been in the hospital longer than I was in our new home, so pulling up to the house did not give me an elated feeling. The home was not very familiar to me after everything I had been through the past six weeks. But I was still determined to remain optimistic.

FINAL STRETCH TO HOME PLATE

Natalia worked nights, and although I was now at home, I was in no condition to watch over myself yet, so *dunt dunt dunt duuh!!* (Superman theme), my older brother Tommy came to the rescue! Tommy was looking for a place to live and since we had a three-bedroom house, and I needed assistance, it was a perfect arrangement. Tommy would now essentially be my babysitter. I'm sure that's how it must have felt at times, him watching me in my wheelchair watching TV.

"Hey Tom, I have to pee, will you grab my urinal?"

I'd pee in the urinal, hand it to him, and he'd dump it in the toilet, and we'd continue talking. The arrangement worked out well. He would get to my place about ten p.m. every night, and Natalia left for work about nine, so that gave me an hour by myself to make sure I didn't fall out of my wheelchair.

One night about two minutes after Natalia left for work, my mind started wandering. *What would I do if I did end up on the ground and I was alone?*

I began looking for my cane, but when I didn't see it immediately, I got nervous. At this point I couldn't imagine trying to walk without my cane. Now I was sitting in my house with my mind racing, because I wanted to be prepared for a worst-case scenario.

"Did you move my cane; I don't see it?"

"Look on your left side." She calmly replied.

"Ha Ha, there it is! Damn you're such a smart girl."

I'd kept forgetting that I couldn't move my left side, and that being blind on the left side thing too. That was the problem though, I kept forgetting it, and that's why the scientists have labeled it left side neglect.

This was not going to be a walk in the park, but hey it was going to get done!

My attitude was the wisest choice I had and complaining could only take me down a dark road, so I laughed, and Natalia eventually made a "game" of it.

The comfy chair I started sitting in after being home for a few days was situated where I watched TV. The hallway was to the left, so Natalia would quietly walk down the hall while I was watching a show.

"Boo!"

She would intentionally scare the crap out of me by grabbing my left arm and get right up on the left side of my face, and either say something or just place her face inches from mine, where I couldn't see her.

These times made it fun. *Damn Natalia,* I felt so damn happy and "normal" in those moments, to just be able to laugh uncontrollably. No thoughts of any of my problems, just my wife and I laughing. I'm so thankful to her, she was my bright shining star, "scaring" me at least once a day.

My sense of hearing had been elevated since the loss of my vision, so every once in a while, her ankle would make that popping sound exposing her. I would look over and she would have her hands over her mouth. She might only have been five feet away and her huge smile would disappear, and she'd laugh and swipe her arm playfully.

"Dang it! I got caught!"

These were honestly some of the best of times during the worst of times.

Even though the therapists trained me on how to get in and out of the shower, I didn't have much confidence in the process. This was yet another thing that was added to Natalia's plate. She would first make sure I got on the shower bench safe, and then I would shower while she went back to her show, or whatever else she wanted to do.

Bang! Bang! Bang!

I'd pound the shower wall with the under-side of my fist as hard as I could, my signal that I was done. Then she would come in to make sure I didn't fall as I got out.

Not a proud time in my life, but I just had to keep my eye on being positive. This shower routine went on for the entire first year. It was just one of those things. My vision was still bad, and I didn't want to misstep on the tile and fall down. This is what I told myself, but maybe there was something more to it. We eventually moved on and came up with new strategies so that I would feel safer. Whatever we did worked because I never did fall.

Hearing the Ping

A few months after the stroke and I hated that I still had to use that (damn) wheelchair. I could walk, but it infuriated me that my pace was so slow. When I went out with a friend or family member for a meal or social event, I just hated the fact that it took me *forever* to get from place to place. In an attempt not to slow them up any more than I already had, I would break down and just use the wheelchair. That was all about to change though.

On a typical Friday afternoon, while sitting in the wheelchair watching TV, I decided to get some fresh air. I wheeled myself to the front door, stood up, and twisted the metal knob with my right hand and opened the heavy oak door.

Dad's words rang in my head and I smiled.

"Location! Location! Location!"

I took in the cute cul-de-sac and all of the greenery that surrounded it, once again reminded that we'd made the best decision when we purchased this home.

Ping Ping Ping!

What I heard was that beautiful sound of an aluminum bat striking a baseball. What I didn't know is that sound would change my life.

"Hey Natalia! Will you please load up my wheelchair and drive me across the street to the baseball field? There's something going on over there!"

"Sure. Are you ready now?"

Natalia drove me over to the baseball field at Arlington High School. After driving through the gate, we ventured down the dirt path that led us to the parking area.

The sight of the green grass and the dirt infield had my soul feeling the best it ever had in the last four months since my life had taken such a drastic turn.

I sat in the passenger seat while Natalia unloaded my wheelchair and wheeled over to my side of the car. I got out of the car and sat in the chair while she made a 180 and popped a wheelie to get us up on the concrete slab where the bleachers were.

As soon as I settled in my spot sandwiched between the Lions dugout on the first base side, and the metal bleachers, I had a feeling of total content. The smell of the grass, the sound of the metal spikes sliding across the concrete floor of the dugout five feet away, and that continuous *ping* created a wonderful and brand-new feeling that I still can't describe. Little did I know, this was so much more than another batting practice of a high school team, it would be my salvation.

The head coach, Gary Rungo, a short stocky man with salt and pepper hair and a matching mustache, was the head varsity coach for the Arlington Lions. He had coached there since the mid-seventies and was quite the legend. I knew of him growing up, and when I got older, I worked for him as an umpire for his summer league games.

"How's it going Donnie?"

In between walking from the field after instructing his players, he stopped by the fence.

"Besides this damn chair? I guess I'm doing pretty good, all things considered."

"Hey Coach! Practice at the same time next week?" One of his players yelled from the chain linked fence.

It was four p.m. and practice was just wrapping up.

"Yes BP, every Friday at three."

"Cool, see you next week coach."

Coach then turned back and looked at me.

"You're welcome to come next Friday, too, Donnie."

His invitation reinvigorated my spirit.

****

The following Friday finally arrived and Natalia dropped me off right before three. I brought my sunflower seeds and my excitement. I had been looking forward to this baseball practice all week.

There was nothing to worry about out there. I didn't have to be concerned with what my wheelchair could or could not do. All that mattered was the sights and sounds of baseball. I had recently recovered most of my senses, so I happily inhaled the smell of the grass and took in everything I could see and hear. There was no other place in the entire world I wanted to be in that moment, under the sun at that baseball field.

All the kids started showing up and started their stretches. Coach approached me by the chain-link fence.

"Hey Donnie. Good to see you. How are you doing?"

Coach Rungo was such a good dude.

"Next Friday we're playing a scrimmage. You should come back. This time you can sit in the dugout."

Let me tell you, that offer put an immediate smile on my face, but it disappeared when I looked down at my wheelchair.

"There's no way I'm going to get into that dugout in this wheelchair!"

It wasn't that I couldn't get the chair into the dugout, but my pride wouldn't allow me to do it.

When I got home that day, Natalia stayed outside with me while I walked ten laps up and down my driveway to work on my pace. I started doing this everyday leading up to the next practice. My mother's walking discipline was rooted inside of me and was starting to take shape.

I would walk down to the sidewalk, turn around and come back up, ten times a day. My neighbors probably either thought I was out of my mind, or very indecisive. I didn't care, I was just determined to walk through the gate, and across the dirt into the dugout, with my cane in hand. That image in my mind made me beyond excited, and I couldn't see anything stopping me at this point. I'm a stubborn guy just like my athletic father. He also had that competitive nature, and I am thankful for that inheritance, too.

I am not a guy who likes to be late for anything, but since Natalia was my ride, I had to be patient. When we drove through the gate, I was disappointed to see that the game had already started. But as luck would have it, one of the assistant coaches, Artie, saw me and opened the gate.

"What inning is it Artie?"

"It's just the top of the first."

He could see this might take me a while, so he kind of guided me around the side of the cinderblock dugout so we could step in. For my safety, the umpire, who stood behind home plate, called time just in case the batter hit a foul ball in my direction. It's a good thing he did, since it would take me awhile to get around the corner to the cover of the dugout. But as soon as my feet hit that concrete of the dugout floor, I felt right at home.

I immediately sat down on the bench with the guys, and put my cane on the ground behind me, out of sight. A bunch of the guys stood at the fence facing the field with their forearms resting at the top of that fence that guarded baseballs from flying inside the dugout.

Just wave hello Donnie!

After a couple of innings, I attempted to talk myself into finding the courage to walk over without my cane in hand. My plan was to lean up against the fence with the other guys. In the bottom of the fourth inning with two outs, I stood up and walked over to an opening between second baseman, Donny Stanford, and his double play partner, shortstop, Bryan Sandoval.

"Hey Donnie, I don't want you to get hit. Please go sit down."

Coach yelled.

Talk about bummed. I sat back down amidst all of the players' chatter in support of their teammates. But all I could think about was how badly I wanted to coach high school baseball.

This is such a beautiful feeling. I feel joy again!

Before that afternoon I wasn't sure I'd feel like that again.

When the ballgame ended, the winner of the game was irrelevant to me, however I felt like the real winner. I felt that Coach Rungo's simple gesture changed my entire path in the most positive way imaginable.

Natalia actually showed up on time. She noticed that once I was settled in the front passenger seat, I was smiling non-stop.

"I can see that you had a good time."

"Oh shit, Natalia, I want to coach high school baseball so bad! But I can't go back to school to get my degree to be a teacher."

It was difficult to talk through the excitement that seemed to be exuding from my pores. I was so giddy.

"Why not?" She responded without blinking.

What was I supposed to tell her? That I wasn't smart enough?

There were a myriad of excuses I surely could have come up with, but instead I just sat there a little in shock. When we pulled up to the house and parked in the garage I went straight to the office and looked up Riverside City College (RCC). I wanted to find out when I could register for classes.

Three days later, Natalia and I headed down to the campus. I filled out the paperwork and got the information about the accommodations available for my visual and cognitive hindrances.

I knew this was something I was interested in and there was no reason to sit around and talk myself out of it. If I spent my days in school, I would be using my brain and working towards something very valuable for my future. Another key to this was that I wouldn't feel like I was a burden on my family. Nobody said anything, but my instincts told me this was the right decision. I'd just have to wait until the fall to start classes.

Now I had more time to get stronger physically, so I began taking longer walks. I started by walking down to the end of the street and back. That was only two houses down, so I would do that multiple times a day.

As my confidence grew, I left the block, and then down to Lincoln which was about one hundred and fifty yards away. I eventually took off to go have lunch at the shopping center that was about half a mile away.

My strength, and confidence were growing by the moment, and both of those things were equally important in my mind. I finally reached the point where I could walk somewhere with someone else and not slow them down to a pace that was outright embarrassing. As I got better and better, I started sitting up each night to brainstorm with myself and set new goals so I could keep improving.

I even came up with a big one. I was going to find a friend that would walk up Mt. Rubidoux with me. This was a famous mountain in Riverside, but the beauty was that there was a paved path to walk up, so this was absolutely something I could do. It was also a goal that would give me a great sense of accomplishment.

Mount Rubidoux has two paved trails that lead to the top where a massive white cross sits. One of the paths has a longer route, which is two miles round trip. The other path is much steeper, just over one mile.

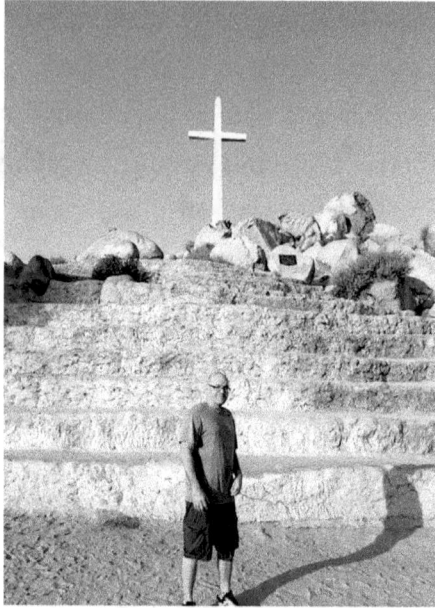

My Dad used to take me and my brothers up there as kids. I actually have a picture of Tom and I sitting on the base of the cross when I was four and he was five. Back then they allowed cars to drive up, but these days hundreds of people walk up the mountain every morning, so that no longer works.

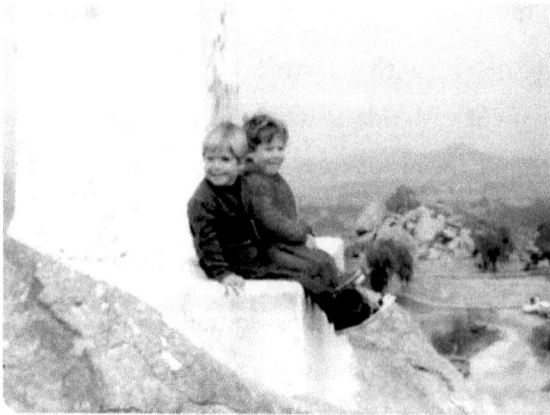

The author and his brother Tom at Mt. Rubidoux. (I'm the cute blonde. Ha Ha!)

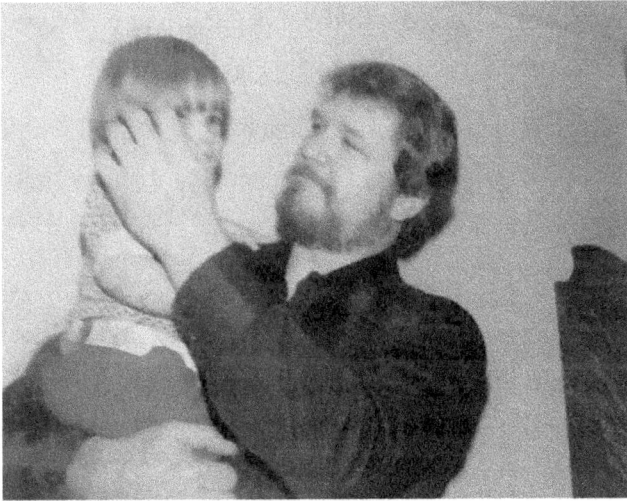

Me and My Dad Joe 1975

It's a great place that attracts all types of people. When I first started walking up Mr. Rubidoux after my stroke, I was motivated by people giving me a thumbs up, when they noticed my limp. After a while, the regulars would recognize me.

"You're doing great Donnie!"

That helped me to keep going.

It was worth it, because when I finally made it to the top, I could see the entire view. Before that I could only see pieces of it when my capacity wouldn't allow me to hike the whole mountain. On a clear day I could see City Hall in the distance, along with many of the older Victorian style homes in the area. I also enjoyed walking up the steep side, because it was more of a challenge.

The picture on the cover of this book was taken up near the top of Mount Rubidoux which gives you some idea of how beautiful the view is.

The first time I made it to the top, I damn near threw a party to celebrate because it was an extremely big deal.

Every Friday at practice, Coach Rungo and I would always discuss my progress. I always had something to share, but nothing was quite as big as when I got to brag that I'd made it to the top of Mount Rubidoux.

With that, he just shook his head with a smirk on his face and invited me to sit in the dugout the following Friday. That was the day his team was playing at Ramona High, the rival school across town.

"Heck yeah coach, I'd love to."

Psyched up all week to be around the game up close again, I got to Ramona a half hour early and anxiously waited for the team to show up. They arrived about twenty minutes before game time. Coach walked with me inside the visitor's dugout and set down his clipboard. He then asked for the guys to huddle around for an important announcement.

"You guys have all been seeing Donnie around a lot. He's been working extremely hard so for now on you can call him Coach Donnie.

He looked at me with a big smile.

"He's our new assistant."

Holy shit, are you serious? Wow, so cool! I fist bumped with Coach Rungo, and to work we went. Since I didn't have a defined role yet, I just kept my eyes and ears open to see how I could assist.

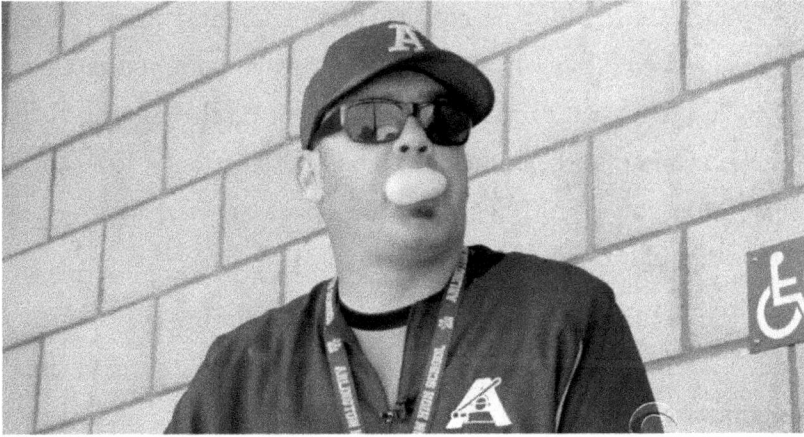

Couldn't be happier. (by Dave Fuller) Photo

It was the top of the first inning, and we had just one out, and Bryce hit a ball into left field that made it to the fence. Our third base coach, Danny, stopped him right there at second base. He was not very fast, so he was happy about that. The next batter hit a hard ground ball that the third baseman had to dive to his right towards the foul line to field. When the third baseman stood up, he saw Bryce was just a few feet from him, so instead of the third baseman throwing the ball to first base to get the batter out, he took one step and tagged Bryce out. That made two outs, and Bryce was not happy. I knew that I needed to talk to him about his base running mistake, especially because his body language clearly let me know he was aware of what he did. He should have made it more difficult for the opposing team to get an out, and with less than two outs and no runner at first base, he didn't need to leave second base until he saw the ball in the outfield to keep him safe.

I waited an inning before approaching him about it, to see if he could shake the frustration on his own. Once I was sure that he had cooled off, I approached him.

"Hey Coop, don't beat yourself up. You know what you did wrong, and you know that with less than two outs, you just have to make sure that the ground ball that is hit on the left side of the infield, makes it to the outfield grass before you attempt to advance, okay? More importantly, don't let this affect you in a negative way for the rest of the game."

He just nodded thanks but didn't give me any eye contact. I knew I was limited in how I could help physically, but my mental toughness was apparent. It became clear to me in that moment that this was the kind of thing that would help me give value to the team. Regardless of Coop's rebuff, I was still on cloud nine. I had gone from being told I might not ever walk again, to walking without a cane! In a dugout of all places! I could not have been happier!

At that game we struck out twelve times as a team, which was far too many, considering that their pitchers weren't that dominant. I went home that night and during my nightly brainstorming, figured out the title for my new role on the team: The Mental Conditioning Coach!

None of the other coaches had my point of view because they had not had the challenges of my recent experience. Knowing what true loss looked like, I could teach the kids about what really mattered, and how key it was to have a strong mindset. It was time to, "get in where I fit in," as the saying goes. Since I obviously wasn't going to be hitting any ground balls anytime soon, I had figured out a new way to play.

Living this new life of mine often made me feel like a little kid. I was constantly keeping my eyes and ears open to whatever advice I could get from anybody that would give me the time. After school each day, the short bus would drop me off at the field. After practice, I would hang around the dugout talking with the other coaches, either asking questions or simply absorbing their conversations.

I hung around the dugout daily. Some of the things I picked up on were much more significant than others. If something I heard stood out to me, I would be sure to ask a question or two to brainstorm on that evening.

I used Ken Ravizza's book *Heads Up Baseball* as my inspiration. My baseball mentor at Riverside City College, Dennis Rogers, used the book as a big part of his curriculum for his class, The Theory of Baseball, Dennis was a mentor to me due to the fact he had teams that won multiple state championships for the RCC Tigers in the early 2000's at the college. I just loved to pick his brilliant brain and was so happy I now had the chance to put all I had learned from him to good use!

That first day of practice after another big loss with excessive strikeouts, I introduced the players to a drill I came up with. This would be something to help increase their success at the plate with two strikes. I took them down to the batting cage in small groups and just let them swing away for the first ten pitches or so.

"Okay the count is one ball and two strikes, so step out of the batter's box, take a deep breath, and have a little self-talk."

I made sure to remind them that they didn't need to try and hit a homerun on the next pitch in the strike zone. It was more important for them to make the opposition have to make a play to get them out. By doing so, the other team would most likely make a lot of mistakes if we as batters put the baseball in play. This would create more success for them, and the team as a whole.

We worked on this drill every week and soon after, we never had more than three strikeouts in one game the entire season. They eventually realized just how important their mental work was in addition to their physical practice.

The second part of my "new play" was meeting up with the guys once a week to study Ken's book aloud. This ritual became known as, "Mental Mondays" as we broke down the book's contents, chapter by chapter, focusing on a different point each week.

Baseball is said to be 90% mental, so it made a lot of sense to me to bring in this angle and give our team a slight advantage in the process. One example was when Boone, our elite lefty, no longer gave up a game tying double in the fifth inning. He adjusted his prior behavior because he became conscious of his body language and his inner thoughts. That way, he was better prepared for the next batter.

The book preaches, "one pitch at a time," and we took that on as best we could. At first, if one of the players swung at a pitch that was clearly in the dirt, he would get mad. But the alternative was to clear his mind, take a deep breath, and move on, one pitch at a time. Coach Rungo gave me freedom to have these meetings, and he himself would come and observe. He saw my value and the great thing was, I did too.

The following season, I was invited back as an assistant. Since I was much better, I asked Coach if I could be the first base coach?

"No, I don't want you to get hurt out there. You're half blind, and I'd hate for you to get hit by a line drive."

But my stubbornness didn't wear off that easily. I brought a base coach's helmet to practice with me the following day.

"Coach get in the batter's box like you're a hitter and hit line drives at me. You'll see that I can see well enough to do this job."

I reached towards the direction that the ball was headed to show him that I saw it. Finally, he hit a hard one just a couple of feet above my head, and I reached up and almost caught it, but it bounced off of the palm of my hand.

"Damn it Donnie, no you're not going to coach first!" He softened putting a hand on my shoulder, "I don't want you to get hurt."

"Come on coach, I just showed you that I saw it."

But he had his mind made up, so I didn't push it. After a year of being around him, I knew he wouldn't budge, so instead of irritating him, I just shut up. After about thirty years of being the head baseball coach at Arlington, he knew what he was doing. I was not about to mess up his routine by being my stubborn self. I had only just begun to learn that sometimes we have to choose our battles, on and off the field.

My second season there, I did find myself doing more instructional stuff on the field. Unfortunately, because of my physical condition, there were instances when I could see in players' eyes that they weren't sure if I knew what I was talking about.

I didn't focus on that, I just kept sharing my knowledge with the boys and eventually gained their trust. They may have been hesitant to take advice from a *diffabled* person who looked different from all their other coaches, but eventually they listened and heeded my lessons. This hesitancy came with the territory, and it was just something extra I had to fight through to accept.

Despite that challenge, I was continuing to have the time of my life! Every day after school I had the short bus drop me off at the field early. I'd go out and walk the bases just to see how fast I could do it. I never felt like I had to take any time off from these personal challenges, because my mind was dead set on how I could improve.

The second season I wore a new brace with an electrical stimulator. There was a little pad underneath my insole at the heel inside my shoe, and the cuff was wrapped around my leg just below the knee. I have what is called foot drop, where my left toes don't move up when I walk and can sometimes almost drag. When I wear the brace, my left heel comes off the ground and sends a message to the brace. This shocks the nerves that are responsible for raising the toes. Wearing this brace did not minimize my sweet limp, but it sure did give me a lot of confidence that I wasn't going to trip while on the field in front of the players. Coach gave me the nickname, "Tenacious D ".

Towards the end of my second season, we learned that the athletic director was planning on implementing a freshman baseball team the following season. Though I may have not been the first, or even second choice for the position, I was the only one who wanted it more than anything. After the first couple of guys the coach asked to fill the position turned it down, I gladly accepted it.

Just think it wasn't long ago that I was sitting in a wheelchair, just wishing I could sit in the dugout! Now look at me!

Now all I had to do was convince fourteen-year-olds with less life experience that a man with a diffability could teach them a few things about the game. I would also do my best to teach them some life lessons while I was at it.

A few of the guys came up to me after practice one day and asked if they could stay and hit in the cages.

Do I stay here and babysit? Or do I see how they can handle themselves?

Since I had plenty of homework, I chose to go work on a class assignment, which in my mind, would give them an opportunity to show me if they could handle themselves or not.

The next day at practice while the team was stretching and warming up, one of the guys came up to me and asked if I had heard what about Jackson and Kay.

"Oh shit, what happened?"

I questioned each player individually to see if all the stories matched up. They were similar, but not exact, and neither one of them were taking the blame. What I learned was that one player got mad at the other, locked him in the batting cage and walked away. About five minutes later, hearing the locked-up players screams, another coach came over and unlocked it.

"Do we have to run now?"

"Absolutely not."

I think of myself as a problem solver, and my punishment for them came to me rather quickly. Since I had been studying communications, I knew at this age they likely hated to speak in public.

"You will both go to the library and find articles on bullying. You will cite five of them in a five-minute presentation in front of the team."

They were pissed, and sad looks came over their faces as they pouted. .

"Can't we just run?"

"No!"

I had never seen any value in asking kids to run as a punishment and I didn't want them to have a negative feeling about that activity. I needed them to see running as a positive part of the sport. They needed to enjoy chasing down fly balls, stealing bases, and hustling down the first base line when they got hit by a pitch, or reached a base safely. With my alternative punishment, I hoped they could learn something new.

Hearing that one of the parents was upset with me, I asked Coach what I should do when he called me that night.

"You gotta deal with it. You're the one that wants to be head coach."

My phone rang again later than evening.

"This is Mrs. Jackson, do you have a minute? I really want to know why my son has the same punishment as the young man who locked him inside the cage?"

"Well, if your son would not have called him fat then he would not have gotten locked in the cage."

"Great point."

When I told the coach about our conversation the next day at practice, he looked at me with a smile.

"That was beautiful."

"Sometimes a simple reason is enough."

"You're a good student Donnie. That school is lucky to have you."

The boys' joint presentation on bullying went well. They also learned that public speaking was not as bad as they once thought. They shook hands, the rest of the team applauded, and we moved on.

My second favorite memory of coaching that freshmen team also had nothing to do with baseball. After Thanksgiving, I asked each student to ask their parents to get them a Target gift card for an amount that might have bought them a piece of clothing that would never leave their closet. They all agreed, and their parents willingly participated.

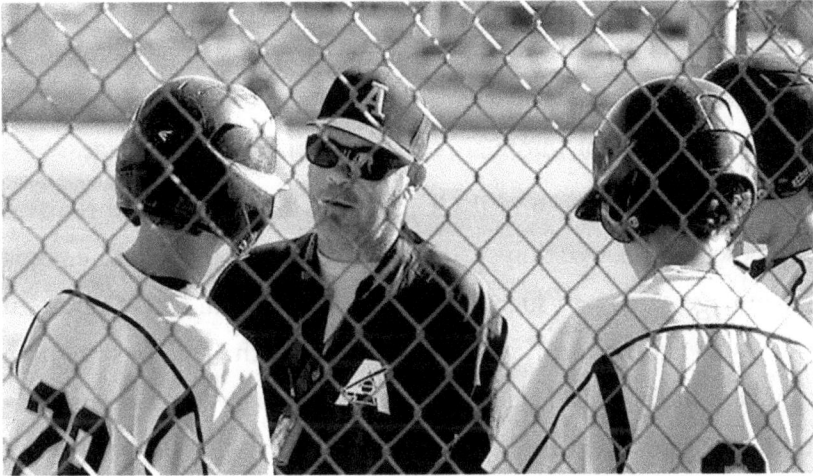

2016 Freshman Baseball Team (Photo by Dave Fuller)

On Christmas Eve, we met up at the local pizza joint for a bite and carpooled to a children's shelter full of teenage runaways. The house mother was so happy to see these unselfish young men, there to give hundreds of dollars in Target gift cards to less fortunate kids. The players stood in the foyer of the group home, filled with excitement as they handed the gift cards to her. Since the group home kids were not allowed to interact directly with them face to face, the house mother thanked them all on their behalf.

They were feeling pretty good about themselves, and for a good reason. Most teenagers are pretty selfish, but these kids learned a good lesson in selflessness. This was a very important seed that I am grateful to have planted.

The cherry on top for me was being invited to City Hall at the end of the year and receiving the Riverside Pride Award for being a positive influence in the city. Most of my team showed up to say a few nice things about me. The fact they did this in front of an audience of strangers affirmed for me that my reason for being their coach extended well beyond baseball. I was so proud of them and their character. They went on to grow up to become wonderful young men, most of whom are currently doing well in college.

I'm not quite sure if Coach ever fully understood that his simple empathetic action of inviting me in the dugout to enjoy a scrimmage game had such an impact on me. I am forever grateful that by including me, he put me on a new path. This was the path that kept me in a good place and allowed me to give back to my community at the same time.

It's nearly impossible for me to feel depressed being around baseball every day. 800,000 Americans have a stroke every year, and 600,000 of those stroke survivors deal with depression according to the Stroke Association. Coach Rungo's kind gesture kept me from being part of that statistic. Things could have been much worse and because of him I had a smile in my soul every day I stepped in that dugout. Another reason my house on Coral Tree couldn't have been in a better location.

Donnie the Student

When I first got to campus, I was full of doubts.

What the heck are you doing? You were a terrible high school student when you graduated twenty-two years ago!

But I quickly flipped my mindset to: *I don't want to depend on my disability check for the rest of my life.*

Becoming a teacher was a career I could do one handed, as well as head coach. I knew if this was truly what I wanted, then I was going to have to dig deep and learn to become a good student. Period!

I also remained determined to do more things for myself to take the burden off of Natalia. One of my big achievements was learning to make a peanut butter and jelly sandwich and put it into a zip-loc bag with one hand. I found inspiration from YouTube videos that featured Nick Vujicic, who was born in Australia without any limbs, but still surfed, swam, and golfed. If he could do it without limbs, I certainly didn't have any excuses! He taught me that I had to avoid using the phrase, "I can't."

My first semester at RCC I was a kinesiology major, and because I had always been involved with athletics, I decided that I would become a physical education teacher.

It took me awhile to get acclimated to being a student again, but when I got two A's during my first semester, my confidence was boosted. I experimented with how many classes I should take per semester, but one of the things I found the most difficult was taking notes and trying to keep up with the professors. I found myself staying after class to ask them questions, which helped when I had even just a sliver of uncertainty. It also built a connection with my professors that lasted well after graduation.

This was the first time I actually had enjoyed school. For once, my classes were my choice, and I felt this was my ticket to freedom and independence. I was more and more determined to not live off of disability checks.

I also proved to myself that I could coach and be successful in school at the same time. By structuring my days with the proper time to study around the baseball practice schedule, I was fine. I wasn't concerned with the fact that it would take me a longer time to finish my Associates degree than most people. I had baseball to fall back on, and by taking two classes at a time, I had more time to spend on the field after I was done with my classes each day.

I hung around the dugout every day after practice, and some of the things I picked up on were much more significant than others, but if it initially sounded significant than I would ask a question or two and then use it as a brainstorming topic later that night.

"It's so difficult to become a high school PE teacher, because those teachers typically stay in those positions longer than other teachers."

DONNIE THE STUDENT

I gave Coach Rungo's words some thought. I didn't want to graduate and have a hard time finding work and knowing Kinesiology was a difficult major, I knew there had to be another way.

My entire life even before my stroke, I had always had empathy and compassion for people with diffabilities, so training to be a Special Education teacher made a lot of sense. I decided to change my concentration to Communication Studies. That would help me as a teacher, a coach, and in life in general.

By the time I had changed my major, I was using some of the accommodations that were available to me, and they really leveled the playing field. (No pun intended.) One of my struggles was finishing my exams in the time frame allotted, because there were many test questions that I'd have to read over ten or fifteen times to understand.

I was growing more and more frustrated, and kept finding myself embarrassed and near tears, because I was struggling so much. Seeing other students getting up and handing the exam to the professor just killed my spirit. But I didn't give up, I spoke up and went to the office for students with diffabilities to tell them of my difficulties. As a result, I was assigned a note taker which helped a great deal. It was also decided that I would take my exams in the disability office, so I'd have double the amount of time to finish them.

Closed mouths don't get fed!

Now I could go to class and just listen and not have to think about anything else! It was such a relief!

I was so grateful for these new adjustments. I no longer had to scramble to get a bunch of notes down before they were all erased which alleviated a great deal of stress.

Some of my fellow students thought I was "lucky," but I assured them the opposite was true.

"Trust me you don't want to trade places with me."

I knew what they meant, and statements like theirs also let me know that things weren't just tough for me, they were tougher. I was grateful for my tutors, especially when they prepared me for my final math exam which was completely stress-free! I was cooler than a frozen lake in Canada and it was a great feeling!

I kept up my work ethic for sixteen weeks, so I didn't have to worry about acing the finals just to pass my class. I worked out a system with my guidance counselor and set up a game plan for what classes I should take and when. I made sure that my schedule was not too demanding and was grateful to the staff who truly looked out for me.

I had my school life together, but my home life was another story.

"Are you okay?"

Natalia was awake which was odd. She always worked until two in the morning, she was usually sound asleep when I woke up in the morning.

"Are you sure?"

"Yes."

I was not convinced, so after asking her a couple more times and getting the same response, I headed out to the living room and had some breakfast. I clearly remember having a gross feeling in the pit of my stomach while I was eating. All I could think about was that amazing woman in the other room. My mind started racing.

Don't go asking her again what is wrong. She may tell you something you don't want to hear!

Being the stubborn guy I am, I did not take my own advice. I marched in our room and sat at the foot of our king-sized bed.

"What's the matter, Natalia?"

She put her hand on my shoulder and sighed as tears rolled down her cheeks.

"I'm sorry Donnie. I can't do this anymore."

I was in total shock.

"No!"

Scared as hell, I went into the living room to sit while my brain ran in circles. *What was I going to do? Where was I going to live? Oh My God! Please tell me this is not really happening!*

After I cooled off, I walked back in the room.

"Is it okay if I stay here until I finish RCC, then figure something out?"

She nodded yes and we managed to maintain an amicable relationship, full of great love and respect. I remain very grateful to her for accommodating me like that.

For the rest of my time living there I concentrated on finishing my studies. I wasn't going to let this impending divorce stop me; I had come way too far.

When her parents invited me over for dinner soon afterwards, I was emotionally shattered. But they welcomed me, showing me great love and compassion regarding the situation. Flo Mamma served me all of my favorite dishes.

"Remember what I told you, Donnie, there is only way out of this family."

"In a box."

I was so relieved to know that they would still consider me family despite everything.

Although it was strange living under the same roof after seven years as man and wife, I was still glad to have Natalia as a friend.

This situation gave me a crash course in strength and maturity for sure, and I still could not bring myself to say the dreaded D word. We didn't argue about it because I accepted her decision. I did not want to be in a relationship if the other person did not. I wanted her to live a happy life, be able to travel like she used to and go on outings with her friends. She had given up so much of what she loved to take care of me and now that I was on the mend, it was her turn to live her life fully and completely. Who could blame her? I was in school chasing my dreams, so why shouldn't she be able to do the same?

I still had my struggles academically, but they didn't stop me, even if I was on the five year plan. I was determined to finish and not have to retake Statistics, like I had heard so many others do! With a tutor's help, I got through it. It was even more difficult than I'd heard about! I channeled my anxiety, and whenever I heard kids talking about their struggles in the class, I encouraged them to seek out the tutor. Believe it or not, I actually ended up leading the study session for the final at my house.

Once again, my mindset saved me. I knew I had to go to the tutor three days a week, discuss the current material, and go over the practice problems. I refused to leave until I could fully explain how to solve the problem. In the end, I earned a very high C grade, proving once again that if I gave a challenge everything I had, I would never go wrong.

Five years after starting at RCC, I finally completed my requirements to transfer. It was a couple of weeks after the 2016 high school baseball season ended, that I graduated with my Associates in Communication studies. I was very proud of myself but also uneasy about the unknown lying ahead.

*****

Now it was time to transfer, and after checking out various schools, and taking a tour of Cal State University of San Bernardino, I found a place that felt like home. Unlike other schools I had visited that seemed a bit snooty, the vibe at CSUSB was filled with hard working students who had not been given anything, just like me.

Since I didn't drive, I decided to live in an apartment on campus so I would have access to everything including the library, my classes, and my professors' offices.

It might have seemed strange for a forty-three-year-old man to be living on campus with a bunch of kids, but it alleviated a lot of unnecessary stress that would've come with the worries of getting to class on time with public transportation.

Although I was proud, I'd made it to a university, my greatest achievement was my independence. Each day I kept in mind that there was a time in my life not long before that when I was unable to put on my own socks. So, the fact that I was going to be living completely on my own was a huge accomplishment for me.

Who would have thought seven years earlier, when my family was being told that I may never walk or talk again, that I'd end up earning two degrees?

I was so grateful to be able to chase after something that brought me so much happiness. I wasn't there to mess around and I made sure everybody knew it. I continued to take my studies very seriously and my new professors soon got used to me occupying their office hours on a

I think word got around that I was much different than the majority of my classmates, most of whom never took advantage of our professors' office hours. One of my professors told me he never saw other students unless they showed up to beg for extra credit, or to give some excuse about a missed assignment.

By the spring quarter of my first year, I found myself either just waving or having conversations in the hallway on the second floor of University Hall with all the professors, whether I was in their class, or not. I was pretty sure that word on the second floor was, "There's an old guy with a limp and a bunch of questions for you if he's in your class." The second floor was where the majority of the Communications offices were located.

By my senior year, professors like Don Girard, who taught Business and Professional Communications, had an office next to my future professor, Dr. Taylor. Dr. Girard knew my name well before I was in his class during my final quarter.

I waited to take my final capstone, the upper division general education courses, until my final quarter. I was very excited to take The World of Islam with Dr. Dany who had won the Golden Apple Award. The award was given to outstanding professors for their excellence in the classroom and their commitment. After I became his student, it was obvious why he had received this award. If a recipient could receive it more than once, I have little doubt he would be in consideration again.

"I am a public servant, and I am here for you."

This was one of his many sayings that revealed his care for his job and his students.

It was easy to understand that there were probably a lot of his students who had preconceived notions about Muslims. I'm sure those ideas practically vanished because of Dr. Dany's peaceful demeanor as a practicing Muslim. He exuded calmness and peace and I can't imagine after being under his tutelage, someone thinking anything negative about him. The fact that he lobbied to create the curriculum for this class in wake of 9/11, was admirable to me.

There were over two hundred students in our class, but he didn't treat anyone like a number. One time a young woman had twisted her ankle and was struggling with pain when she walked. Dr. Dany called security to come with a golf cart to help her get to her car. This is just one small example of how he showed his care for people in general. He was a great role model, especially to me.

I was always the last student to leave his class. I would sit there at my desk after the two-hour lecture, waiting for the line of my fellow students to end. After speaking to the last student in a line that had formed at his podium, he made his way over to me. He knew I would always have at least one question regarding that evening's lecture.

I was dedicated to doing well in all of my classes, but I must admit there was a little bigger push when this professor showed so much respect to everyone he came in contact with. His commitment made me determined to show him how hard I was going to work for him and how much I cared about him, too. I was ecstatic when I got an A on his first midterm exam because it proved that my effort was paying off.

I honestly don't feel that college is that hard. All one has to do is complete the given assignments with great effort, follow directions, and hand them in.

I could have easily hit the snooze button every morning, but instead, I woke up at six a.m. regardless of whether my first class was in the morning or the afternoon. Each day, I made sure to have a solid breakfast and I got to work. I treated school like a full time job, the same way I had treated my recovery from my stroke.

I had looked at my ability to be back in school at my age as a blessing, and nothing to ever be taken for granted. I couldn't go back to bartending because I was no longer able to perform those job duties. I still considered myself lucky. If someone else my age woke up tomorrow and decided that he just hated his job and wanted to enroll in school to chase his passion, it would be a lot tougher. If they had kids and needed to work to bring in enough income to support their family, they would not have the freedom I did.

I had no kids and was on disability. I was glad that given my situation, I was in a place financially where I had the privilege of chasing my dreams.

What separated me from the majority of my fellow students was the procrastination factor. As soon as I received a group assignment, I was ready to jump on it right away. Most of my fellow students would want to wait until the last minute, but I would encourage them not to. I would get everyone together and they would eventually cooperate. That way, we could finish the first version, and spend the rest of the time making adjustments. We were fully prepared, while the other groups ran around and stressed out, trying to figure out how they would finish on time.

My work ethic continued earning me good grades. In addition, I never missed a single day of class, or walked in late. I never turned in an assignment late or failed to turn one in altogether, like I did in high school. This routine helped keep my stress level down, and that mattered a great deal to me.

Most of my challenges had nothing to do with my *diffability*. As an older student I had a lot of life experience, which was probably my greatest advantage, While their advantage over me was that they were much more tech savvy. I usually got a chuckle out of them after telling them I graduated from high school before the internet was invented. I had never been a fan of this new technology, and now with the loss of much of my vision, it just compounded the problem for me, especially for our group assignments.

After a while, I would simply identify who was good with PowerPoint and get tips from that person. With practice, I eventually got better at it.

As the days got closer to the end of college, I started visualizing myself in my graduation gown walking across the stage to receive my diploma. I was really starting to get excited. Boy, this has been a long journey!

But as my time at CSUSB was winding down, I realized that I just didn't have a burning desire to be a teacher any longer. I was still periodically showing up in Riverside to volunteer in a local special education class, but it wasn't giving me the feeling it used to.

What the heck was I going to do? I had just spent seven years in school and now I was changing the entire plan?

I had also been volunteering as an inspirational speaker at Ballard Rehabilitation Hospital. I had been going there on the third Tuesday of the month to speak to the new stroke patients since 2011. I did this because after my stroke, I had always wanted to talk to someone who had been through what I was going through. My doctors and therapists had a lot of book knowledge, but none of it was firsthand.

I never found that person to talk to, so I decided to become that person. After I worked my butt off and got myself physically and mentally in a position to go back to school, I asked the head staff at Ballard if I could come in once a month. I wanted to speak to the stroke support group and give some encouragement with a perspective they could relate to.

I fell in love with speaking and have been doing it for over a decade. Ironically enough, I have only spoken to a handful of individuals that were physically as bad off as I was when I was there. For them to be able to hear the testimony from my former nurses, and to see me today, offers them great encouragement. That is why I do what I do, to see the look on their faces that lets me know they know they can overcome their stroke, and live full lives just like I have.

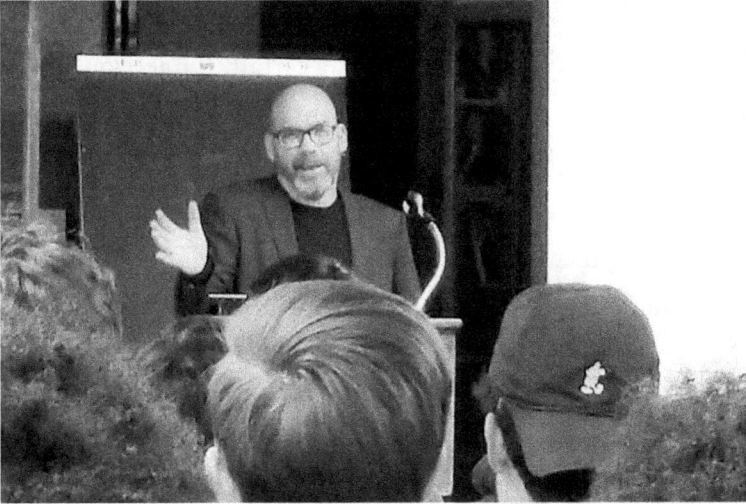

Speaking to the RCC Track and Field Team for Coach McCarron.

On December 8, 2018, I got the privilege of walking across the stage in the Coussoulis Arena at Cal-State University of San Bernardino, to receive the bachelor's degree that I had worked so hard for.

"No matter what happens in your life, how much money you earn, or how much debt you go into, nobody can ever take your education away from you."

I remembered the words of my Sports Psychology professor Jim McCarron back at RCC and smiled at myself at that profound statement he made one afternoon.

I absolutely love the game of baseball, and I love teaching as well, but the more I recovered, the clearer it became to me that I could do even more.

Now with my degree in hand, the initial plan of why I wanted to earn it was gone. But I didn't feel like I had wasted any time, I knew my education was invaluable.

The best thing happened to me during my final quarter. I saw a young man named Austin who I felt a certain connection with. He couldn't have been older than twenty-three. He walked around dragging his feet with his arms which were slid inside forearm crutches. Each time I saw him I felt sorry and inspired by him at the same time. When I met him, I learned he had cerebral palsy. I had often gotten rides around campus in a golf cart. But after seeing his resilience, I stopped. *If that guy was walking, I could, too.*

We had another very special connection.

"Do you like baseball?"

He went silent for a moment.

"I love baseball."

That led to my telling him about my campus radio show, "Donnie's Dugout." And ironically enough, he had been scheduled to volunteer in the station that quarter. To make a long story short, Austin ended up being my on-air broadcast partner.

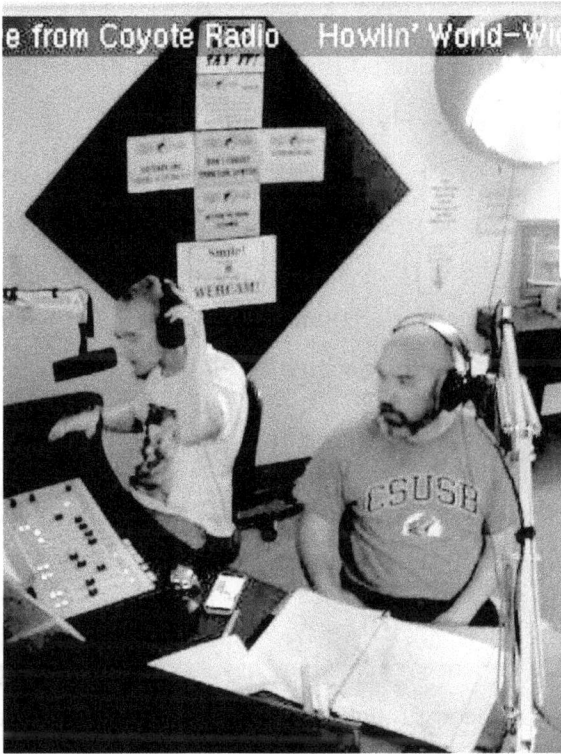

Donnie's Dugout with Austin on Coyote Radio

Baseball players are known for having nicknames, and because of all of the things I thought of Austin before we met, I gave him the nickname, "Nails."

"Austin, you are tough as nails!"

Nails and I would meet up for lunch in the commons on Monday and put together our lineup. The lineup consisted of nine topics of discussion that happened the previous week in baseball.

We enjoyed bantering about Jose Altuve who I was a big fan of. We would discuss how important that 5'3" man was to the Houston Astros, and baseball as a whole. Austin called this "inning" the Altuve love fest. He enjoyed giving me a hard time.

Nails had a voice for radio for sure and did a great job with changing his inflection and tone. He teased me by telling me that I had more of a face for radio.

It was a great way to end to my college career by working with him, the same young man that I used to look at from afar admiring his toughness. By refusing to give excuses, he challenged me. I still have a lot of respect for that dude. Before meeting him, I just wanted to walk over and give him a high five for being so resilient. I knew that most people in his situation would never put themselves in such a vulnerable position. By thrusting himself on campus around thousands of others in his age group, he showed strength and courage. Most of his peers would have never dared to do this if their roles were reversed.

From a distance, people may have seen a man struggling. The reality was that he was much more secure in his situation than I was.

Perspective, perspective, perspective.

I could walk at least three times as fast and hold an umbrella with my right hand during a rainy day. Even though he couldn't do either one, it didn't matter to him. He kept a positive attitude and did his best, which was pretty damn great!

I had always seen myself as mentally tough, but this guy was the king. I was and am so thankful that we got to spend so much time together. He taught me so much more than some of my professors did.

Before my graduation ceremony, I had watched many YouTube videos of past commencement ceremonies from CSUSB and imagined myself getting my degree. It was even better than I had imagined. I even got to sit next to Louis and Jasleen, two of my favorite classmates.

When the time came for our row to stand up and head to the stage, I heard my name being yelled from those bleachers. I slowed down just a touch to see who it was that was calling out my name.

I looked over to see my mom standing up trying to take a picture of me.

"Donnie! Stop so I can take a picture!"

There was a stampede of graduates behind me, so that was not an option. As I got closer to the stage, the feeling in my stomach felt like anxiety on steroids. This was so cool!

All of the assignments I completed, and all of the exams I had to pass to get to that stage could have seemed insurmountable...But now I got to tell people that I graduated with the highest GPA in the history of the school!

I was now a proud member of Lambda PI ETA honor society for the discipline of Communication Studies.

When I would tell people that my cumulative GPA was a 6.4 they would shake their heads.

"How is that possible?"

"Well think of it like this, if you had a 4.0 it would probably seem reasonable to attribute a 2.0 to each side of your brain, right? Well, I only have one side, so I take my 3.2 and multiply it by 2."

That seems fair to me, and it's still always good for a chuckle.

I got myself up the stairs and reached the stage and looked out across the sea of people. After I received my degree, I headed back down and the first person I saw was Dr. Dany who greeted me with a congratulatory hug.

"Let's take a selfie."

I now have that photo hanging in the entryway of my apartment.

I saw my Mom in the bleachers but didn't see Xavier or my middle school friend, Jeremy (AKA "Peaches"), until after my name was called.

I most definitely wanted to have a party to celebrate but decided to have it on Sunday, so my party would not compete with my classmates. I wanted them to celebrate with me. It was a fun time and two of my professors from RCC even showed up, along with one of my favorite communication professors from CSUSB.

What a monumental lesson I learned through this whole process. We cannot let others tell us what we are capable of. Nothing, let me repeat, nothing is a guarantee, but instead it seems that everything is to be determined.

My realization of this came to me while I was on a walk on Christmas Day, just a few weeks later when I was walking up a semi-busy road.

Donnie you just have to get to that telephone pole, and you can turn around.

The telephone pole was only about twenty yards in front of me and it was raining. A large truck passed me from behind

If that driver had been looking down at their cell phone for even a brief moment, they could've veered off the road and ran me over.

It was yet another reminder that I couldn't afford to take anything for granted. Even though I could see that telephone pole, and walked nearly a mile to that point, there was still no guarantee that I would make it.

As soon as I did, I touched it and turned around to head back home. Wouldn't you know it! The first car that drove past me slammed on their brakes and slid within one foot of the pole I had just touched.

May my perspective keep me humble.

CHAPTER 12

Donnie the Graduate

Now that I was a new college graduate at the age of forty-five, I had to move off campus. I found a one-bedroom apartment at a place called The Aspens. When I was in high school, my friends and I considered these the *cool* apartments. It was a beautiful place, with a massive number of tall trees along with a couple of ponds filled with koi fish and turtles. One of my favorite aspects of living at The Aspens was that right outside my patio window, was the bus stop.

There is no other apartment complex like this in Riverside and moving there was a great accomplishment for me.

A few of my good friends helped get me moved in. Keys in hand, IKEA furniture in place, music hooked up to Pandora *and* my friends? This was a new kind of heaven.

"I DID IT!"

A tear of joy escaped from the corner of my right eye as I reached up towards the sky.

All that had happened: marriage, the purchase of a home, the stroke, coaching the guys, the divorce, my college degrees, and now I was independent enough to live on my own! I had made it! Despite this reality, there were plenty of days that it all seemed like a dream.

In September 2009, I was told I would probably never walk again. In 2018, nearly a decade later, I walked into my new apartment. This was all in the same week that I walked across the stage as a college graduate!

Without a job right after graduation, I found myself for the first time in seven years, with no schoolwork. It was thrilling to be able to jump on the bus most days to just get out and visit with people.

I had gotten trained through the bus company on how to get around, and this training was available to me because I was a former user of Dial-A-Ride, a bus service for people with diffabilities. Because of the training I received, I also was eligible for a free bus pass. With all of this time on my hands, I now had the freedom to jump on a bus whenever I needed to go anywhere. The feeling of independence I now had was priceless.

Another reason I was so excited is because the week I moved into the Aspens, I was also prescribed a CGM by Dexcom. CGM is the acronym for Continuous Glucose Monitor. When I was diagnosed with Diabetes in 1980, my glucose could only be checked by dipping a strip into a cup of urine and matching the color on the strip to the color on the strip bottle. Back then I had to do all of that just to get a ballpark of my blood sugar level. As time went on, I had to prick my finger and put a blood sample on a strip that was inserted into a blood glucose monitor.

Technology has sure proved itself in science because I now have a monitor inserted in my abdomen that checks my glucose level every five minutes. It is connected with the Bluetooth on my phone. If my glucose gets too high or too low, my phone will alert me. This is the best because it allows me to live on my own, and if my sugar is low and I need help, I get it automatically.

The loud beeping has woken me up in the middle of the night a handful of times in the last year and a half, but I am happy that my former diabetes life is a thing of the past.

When I first arrived at Ballard, my doctor asked me if I knew I was diabetic because my A1C (average of glucose readings over a period of time) was at an extremely high 15. Last time I checked, it was a 5.9. Although 7 is considered perfect, I'm satisfied with my current number.

"Donnie, you're doing great! Just relax."

My endocrinologist is always telling me I'm doing fine but I still remain extra vigilant of my number, my diet, and exercising.

This CGM has turned me into a control freak and I am always asking Siri what my number is. If she responds with a number I don't like, near 200 or above, I then stop and reflect on how much insulin I gave myself for my last meal. How cool is that? It's amazing as far as I'm concerned.

The CGM has to be changed out every ten days, but overall, it's been a great help for me to keep my diabetes under serious control.

****

When visitors step into my home they will immediately notice a wall with a line-up of photographs of my family, Dr. Dany and me on my graduation day, and my college diploma in a 16 x 20 frame.

These are evidence of a long mountain that I have climbed my entire life. They represent hard work, heartbreak, and accomplishment. These photos represent obstacles both physical and mental, that I have conquered. My new goal now was to keep climbing. There is always another goal to set. Just start at the end of your driveway.

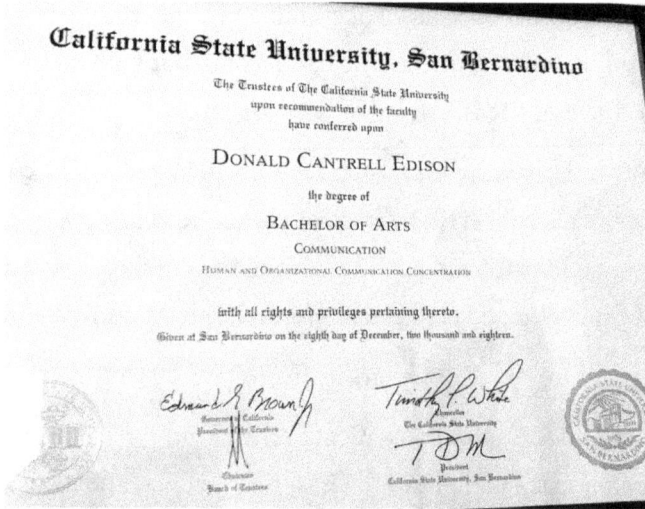

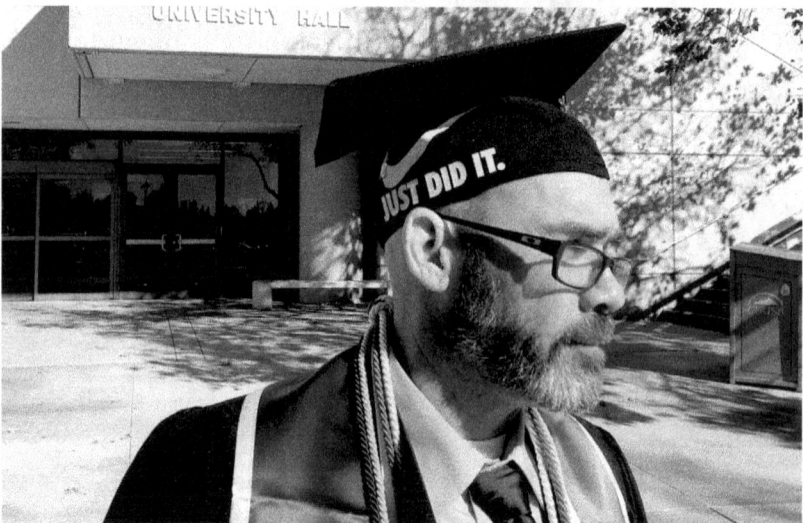

Check the 'Just Did It"

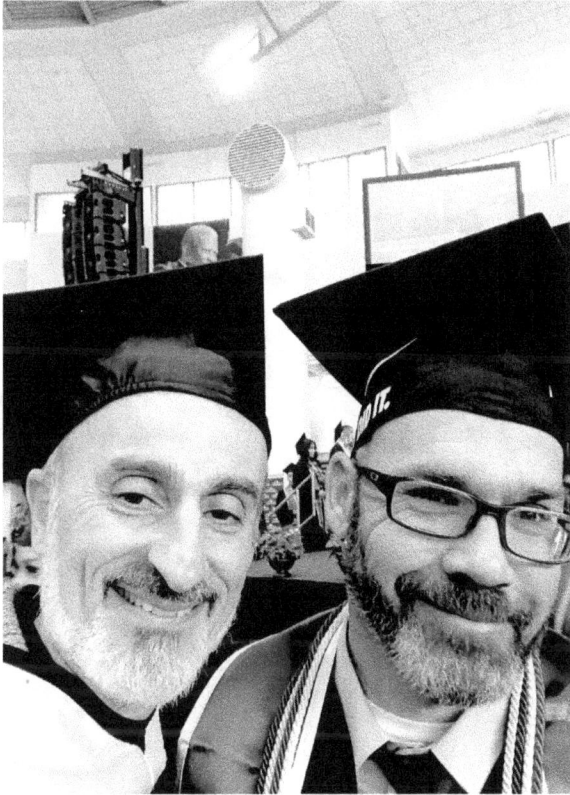

Photo By, Dr. Dany (Coolest Professor on Campus)

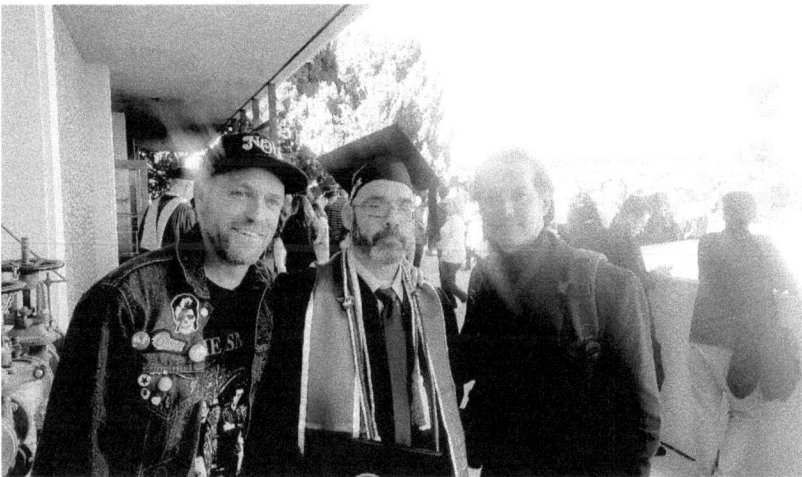

Jeremy (Peach), Me, Xavier. High School Buddies.

CHAPTER 13

New Perspectives

Perspectives, we all have them, and while writing this book I have come to realize that they are continuously changing in correlation with our life experiences. One example that stands out is that I used to hope I would never have to use a city bus in my adult life after owning a car. But today, I couldn't be more grateful that I have the ability to walk out to the bus stop and go where I need to.

I remember the day Natalia and I got the keys to our new home and hoping I would never have to live in an apartment again. But today, I am not only grateful to live in an apartment, I am glad I can afford to stay here. By keeping an open and accepting mind, I have prevented myself from being miserable and depressed. I could have easily chosen to talk myself into believing I was a failure because of it.

My friend, Pete, continued to teach me a valuable lesson. I kept my promise and Natalia and I would visit him at their home in

Moreno Valley. Shortly after his release from Ballard, he had another stroke and continued to deteriorate. Eventually a hospital bed was put in their living room, and I can't begin to explain how hard it was to see him like that. I'm sure it was that much more difficult for Nadia who would soon be a widow.

In the end, he was completely bedridden, and I doubt he even knew we were there. It was a sad time, but I remain grateful for the memories of our animated conversations at Ballard. God bless you, Pete Pederson!

When Natalia decided to go a different direction, it made sense for me to have a response that would keep me on track. It wasn't easy, but I was on a mission. It was 100% worth it to realize that I needed to come up with a game plan for my mindset to finish school and not be sidetracked by our impending divorce.

I remember the first few days being excruciatingly painful, but that   was because of my subconscious. I knew that I loved her, but on the other hand, I wasn't going to beg her to stay married to me. Feeling as lost as I did in the initial days and weeks afterwards, I responded to the situation by respecting her wishes, despite my hurt feelings. Because I did, we still have our bond, which I am beyond thankful for. It hurts to see friends of mine divorce on bad terms, and I am glad that I avoided that outcome.

I am further strengthened knowing that despite the fact that the World Health Organization, (WHO) reported that 2.2 million deaths were attributable to high glucose problems to Diabetics in 2012, that I was not one of them.

The people that are part of that death statistic did not take care of themselves and died as a result. The way I see it, if I hadn't had my stroke, I would have had an extremely high chance of dying from high glucose complications just like they did. The way I was eating and drinking before the stroke kept my glucose levels on the high end. It is absolutely remarkable that as badly as I treated my body, I had no serious episodes and somehow maintained a low glucose level. The fact that my donut lunches in high school, and bad habits that continued into my adulthood didn't kill me, makes me unique. My stroke was my wakeup call and I know for a fact that I am one exception of millions, and I don't take any of that for granted.

I hope my message was received well. I want you, the reader, to know that at some point in each of our lives we will get knocked down or turned upside down like mine was. We will see it happen to our friends, family, and loved ones, too. I want you to remember that although we don't choose the bad things that happen to us, we do get to choose how we respond.

My theory is that whether people come out of an awful experience or don't make it at all, depends on them to a large extent. The attitude we choose to respond with, makes all of the difference. If I had given up, I would probably never have walked again, much less gotten a degree or become a coach! How people come out of a tragedy, all boils down to the attitude they chose to respond to it with.

The response is everything!

No matter how bad things seem, there is always a bright side if we look hard enough.

So even though life has brought us challenges both before and after COVID-19, it brings us blessings, too. This is where our focus needs to be. Despite the storms that we are forced to go through in life, we must keep seeking the sun. By doing so, we will not only have a happier outcome, we will find a greater love and respect for ourselves.

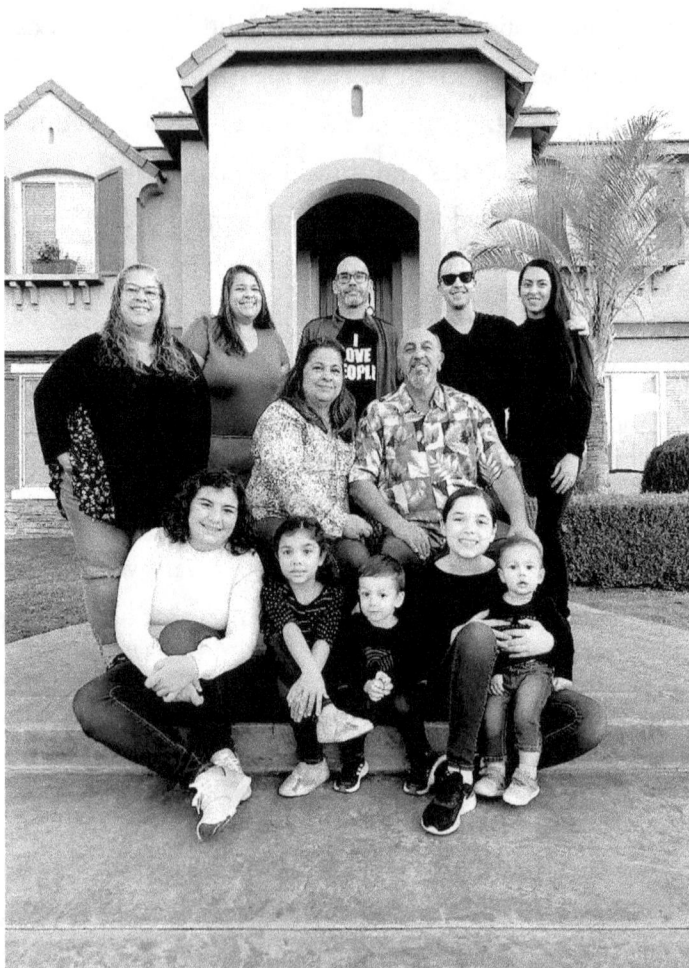

Front Row: Callie, Ella, Emerson, Sophia, and Harrison
Middle Row: Flo and Amir
Back Row: Mercedes, Natalia, Donnie, Joe, and Monica

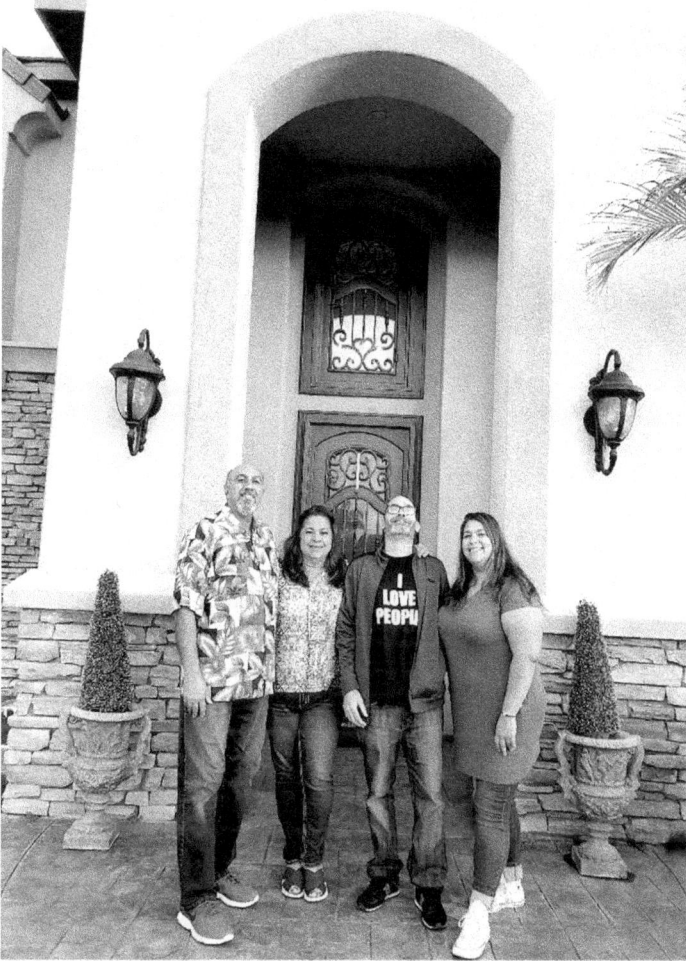

Dad, Mom, Donnie, and Natalia

Epilogue

On my bedroom wall is a picture of Natalia at the age of six. This photo makes my face and heart smile every time I look at it. Amir told me that a couple of days before the picture was taken, she had fallen and knocked out her two front teeth, which is why she has a gap in the front. Her hair is cut in a cute mullet style. How could I not smile every time I walk by that photo?

"Look at that little face, that cute little face."

Natalia visits and she still just thinks I'm silly for having that photo and talking to it. She remains my favorite person in the entire world, and that picture makes me happy, so I leave it right where it is.

I'm happy that we have remained great friends with great respect for one another. I know that doesn't happen in a lot of cases of divorced couples.

Natalia has worked her way up and is now working on private yachts as a chef. She gets to travel the world and make a living doing it, and she just loves it. This is a great example of why I still have so much love for the woman who I once called my wife. I am so grateful to have such a close connection with this amazing human being.

"Donnie, just so you know when I talk to people about you, I don't refer to you as my ex-husband, I refer to you as my best friend. I do that because my ex-husband doesn't sound like we are still in each other's lives."

Damn it, I love her so much! What a woman! We still laugh and joke with each other, and even call each other, "Kid" in text messages. I always spend my holidays with Flo Mamma and Amir and they are always there for me. They have been surrogate parents to me, especially after my mom passed away, and I love them so much.

When COVID-19 hit the United States in March 2020, I stopped taking the bus. If I need to go to the grocery store Amir takes me. I sure miss getting out and about each day, but this was the adjustment I needed. Living on my own and not being able to get out and socialize has gotten tougher and tougher as the months have rolled on by.

We all have noticed how this quarantine has slowed our lives down and forced us to take care of things we had neglected before, especially our loved ones. We could focus on all of the so-called negatives or take the time to list all of the positive things.

With all I have been through since my stroke, I know it could be so much worse, so I simply choose to remain grateful.

Today I live in a new apartment. Though it is not as nice as The Aspens was, and my finances aren't exactly where I'd like them, I still have a lot of hope.

EPILOGUE

In 2019, a doctor signed a document that labeled me as TBD, which doesn't stand for "To Be Determined". It means that I am totally and permanently disabled. This label defers my student loans, meaning if I can't work for the next three years then I will no longer have to pay them back. That is a sigh of relief when a guy can't work and he has debt. But no matter what, I am still on the hunt for something I can do for a living so I can pay them back.

I have also ramped up my morning walking routine and am now walking 4.5 miles each morning. My next goal I've set is to walk the LA Marathon before I turn 50. I have three more years to go!

By continuously setting goals, I have found this to be a great way of keeping my mind excited about something, while simultaneously improving my physical self.

I recently re-watched a clip on YouTube of the interview that Steve Hartman did with me for his show on CBS, "On The Road". I say something that may seem ridiculous when you first hear it.

"I am thankful for my stroke."

One might think that I didn't mean that. But the point I was making was that my mindset was embedded in seeking the good. It would not have served me or my recovery to rant and rave about how much the stroke disrupted my life.

I have also been known to say that I am grateful that the stroke happened when I was thirty-six, and not seventy-six. At thirty-six, I knew I had a better chance of recovering, because I was younger. Pete Pederson definitely taught me that.

I am even more grateful when I take into account this fact:

According to The World Health Organization, 2.2 million

deaths were attributable to high glucose problems to Diabetics in 2012. These are people who did not take care of themselves and died as a result. The way I see it, if I hadn't had the stroke, I would have had an extremely high chance of dying from high glucose complications just like they did. The way I was eating and drinking before the stroke without monitoring myself properly, kept my glucose levels on the high end. It is absolutely remarkable that as badly I treated my body, I had no serious episodes and survived when so many others did not. The fact that my donut lunches in high school, and bad habits that continued into my adulthood didn't kill me, made me a rare exception. My stroke was my wakeup call and I know for a fact that I am one fortunate guy. So many millions didn't make it, and I refuse to take that fact for granted.

My goal is to live a happy life and so that is what I strive to do.

So, when you find yourself in a tough situation, make sure to stop and consider the things in your life that make your soul smile. Immerse yourself in those things whether they are people, hobbies, or your favorite book.

I am living proof that focusing on what makes you happy works and if you have the right attitude, the sun will always appear after the storm.

Thank you for your support.
To contact Donnie about speaking at your
event, school or rehabilitation center, email

donniespeaks@yahoo.com

Follow Donnie at:
@DonnieSpeaks   @DonnieEdison

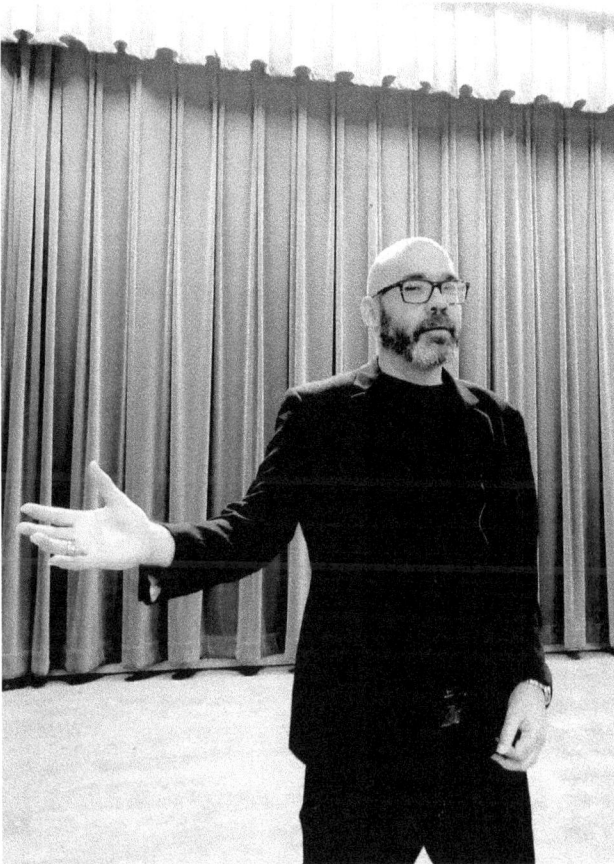

www.ingramcontent.com/pod-product-compliance
Lightning Source LLC
Chambersburg PA
CBHW052208270326
41931CB00011B/2267